VITAMIN C: HOW BEST TO USE IT

HOW IMPROPER CLINICAL TRIALS HAVE MISLED US!

Second Edition

Separating fact from fiction to ensure proper use

Stephen Sheffrey, D.D.S.

SERVICE PRESS
Box 130104
Ann Arbor, Mi 48113

Publisher's Cataloging-in-Publication
(Provided by Quality Books, Inc.)

Sheffrey, Stephen.
   Vitamin C : how best to use it : how improper
clinical trials have misled us! : separating fact from
fiction to ensure proper use / Stephen Sheffrey. -- 2nd
ed.
   p. cm.
   Includes bibliographical references and index.
   LCCN: 2001126876
   ISBN: 0-9629372-3-1

   1. Vitamin C. 2. Vitamin therapy. 3. Orthomolecular
therapy.   I. Title.

RM666.A79S48 2001   615'.328
                             QBI01-201220

VITAMIN C: HOW BEST TO USE IT

Second Edition

CONTENTS

*The letter C first represented the "antiscurvy factor" in 1918 when experimental rat food containing the factor was labeled the C diet. In 1920 it became vitamin C. Its pure form was isolated from cattle adrenal glands by Albert Szent-Gyorgyi (1928). Thinking it was a new type of sugar but ignorant of its formula, he proposed naming it **ignose**. (The names of sugars end in ose.) A journal editor vetoed the flippancy; and **godnose** also. They agreed to name it **hexuronic acid**. It was reported to be the long-sought pure form of vitamin C in 1932. In 1933 Szent-Gyorgyi changed its name to **ascorbic acid**. In 1934 the American Medical Association's Council on Pharmacy and Chemistry decided the name suggested it was therapeutic, therefore was promotional, a no-no if a substance was to be included in AMA publications. In the January 5, 1935 issue of the AMA Journal the council advised that the term **cevitamic acid** be used in AMA publications. But scientists in Europe where most of the research was being done continued to use the term **ascorbic acid**. In 1939 the Council faced reality, junked its term and allowed **ascorbic acid** to be used in AMA publications.*

If not available in stores, this book can be ordered at $4.95 (U.S.) from Service Press, Box 130104, Ann Arbor, MI 48113. Shipped postpaid in U.S. (book rate). Add $2.50 if Priority-Mail shipping is desired. No shipping in November and December. No shipping after October 2005.

Introduction

Critics say that advocates of higher vitamin C intake are orbiting a distant planet. Advocates say the benefits are applicable here on earth. When collected in one chapter they're quite impressive. The rare serious side effects are impressive also to the few who are at risk. Those hazards are discussed in detail so they can be avoided.

The hazard everyone faces lies in the misinformation about C. In April, 2000, authorities recommended an adult RDA of 75 mg for women and 90 for men, a rise from the previous 60 mg. After reading this book you may consider the amount to be about like the minimum wage---okay for young teens but not enough for older folks to live well on.

The authorities also advised an upper intake limit of 2,000 mg daily. And of course it was claimed the vitamin can't prevent colds. Surely they were aware that even the inadequate doses used in well done scientific trials did prevent colds in a few individuals, a seldom mentioned fact. As for an upper limit of 2,000 mg a day, experienced users would consider it about the right limit every 30 minutes while treating influenza.

High-dose advocates rate those authorities as either grossly uninformed or engaged in an ongoing effort to mislead the public. The public would be better informed by the statement that marketing strategy for prescription drugs be considered whenever negative statements are uttered about vitamin C. The first four chapters should convince even innocent critics that certain important scientific trials were designed to discredit the vitamin, not to prove its value.

If it ever comes to pass that objective clinical trials are conducted with oral or intravenous C in its therapeutic dose range, it will be seen that it is as much a miracle drug as those created in laboratories.

1

VITAMIN C: HOW BEST TO USE IT

Bias Against Low-tech Medicine Is Hazardous To Your Health

Before discussing how best to use vitamin C, the subtitle of this book, *How Improper Clinical Trials Have Misled Us,* should be justified. An excursion into that area will also impart a better understanding of the nature of the vitamin.

We'll start with a look at two medical cases, one of which occurred forty years before the other. Case WC: A physician in his sixties writhed in pain from a debilitating bout with shingles. In spite of the best care his doctor knew how to provide, the disease did not subside for a month. A side effect of one of the drugs prescribed dropped the patient into spells of weeping, moods entirely foreign to his normally unflappable nature. He never fully recovered. He was left with an altered gait and the need to take medication to ease the residual pain that afflicts a good percentage of those who've had the disease. I'm well acquainted with the details of this case; the patient was a good friend.

Case DS: A man, 65, doubled over in pain, shuffled into his doctor's office. At first glance the doctor suspected an internal problem that suggested a need for surgery. Then he saw the typical picture of shingles on the man's abdomen. The doctor injected an intravenous solution containing 3 grams of an antiviral substance and told the man to return in 4 or 5 hours for another injection. He returned in 4 hours, free of all pain. By the next day the wide strip of blisters had begun to dry up. A few more injections cleared the disease in 3 days, a wondrously quick result for such a severe case. Phenomenal---yet just a routine cure of shingles by the doctor.[1]

Great! you may be thinking, *miraculous medical progress in forty years!* The advances in pharmaceutical chemistry during that time are almost unbelievable and deserve our considerable admiration. The sequence of these cases was reversed, however. The last one described---the speedy cure of shingles---*occurred forty years before the first one!* Since that time thousands of patients with shingles have suffered mightily with the disease and its aftereffects simply because most physicians are unaware of the low-tech antiviral substance the doctor injected.

What is the substance? Sodium ascorbate, an injectable form of vitamin C.

High-dose C was shown to be effective against shingles prior to 1936, when the former Chief of Dermatology at University of Geneva published his first batch of case histories. He predicted that C would be the future medicine of choice for shingles, as well as for oral and genital herpes.[2]

Why isn't it, then? Why did a remarkable nontoxic cure, which hasn't yet been surpassed by better therapy, fail to become the medicine of choice for shingles and herpes, as predicted in 1936?

A look at the recent history of the vitamin suggests an answer: After C was made synthetically in 1933 it became plentiful---and pure, so that scientists knew what they were working with. They soon confirmed that it has antiviral and antitoxic properties. Citing 18 references to published papers, a scientist wrote in 1937 that it had inactivated every virus and toxin which was investigated. And added that therapeutic results with diphtheria and tuberculosis were outstanding.[3] [Diphtheria is in a sense a viral disease; the strain which is so toxic is infected with a virus.]

Encouraging research reports prompted Merck to promote its brand of C for fevers and infections via a full-page ad in the December 17, 1938 issue of the AMA Journal. By that time a 10-gram dose [10,000 milligrams] had been given intravenously; and gram doses had been given daily for months.[4] Extra C was seen to reduce dramatically the number of sick days due to common diseases, including whooping cough.

By the late 1930s the vitamin was on its way to becoming a major therapeutic drug.

But not for long. Second thoughts were brewing. Vitamin C was not a prescription item and not patentable. It was not a highly profitable product and because anyone could buy it, quacks were touting it and other vitamins as cure-alls. To some doctors, treating with a quack medicine was demeaning. Also, they could not judge the effectiveness of their own therapies if the patients were doping themselves with extra C as well. The vitamin was becoming a nuisance.

Another problem doctors had with extra C is that about 1 in 5 patients cannot take oral doses high enough to be effective. Although nearly everyone can tolerate large amounts given by injection, about 20% of those who try high doses orally experience distressing side effects such as intestinal gas, cramps, diarrhea, mouth irritation or a light rash. Patients did not want to take another dose of such medication.

As for the 80% who *can* take enough C orally to subdue viruses, the benefit is elusive if it is not taken properly. And in the 1930s proper dosing was partly a lucky guess. Back then, so many confusing doctor reports of experience with C appeared that an authority stated: "Out of the work already reported (50 to 100 articles per month for the past 3 years) has emerged a mass of material made up of truths, errors and debatable questions of which the last mentioned group constitutes the major portion."[4]

The above statement was written in 1938. It could very well apply today. Errors and debatable questions still encumber many scientific trials; doses are seldom tailored to the individual; participants are not checked for sensitivity, so that trials include those who cannot tolerate effective doses; more C is absorbed when taken with citrus juice after fatty food but this knowledge is ignored; the blood level of the vitamin is not kept consistently high because the span between doses exceeds 3 hours; and the doses used are too low anyway.

In addition to inadequate dosing, most of today's information about C is gathered from trials in which participants are *healthy*, not sick. It's like testing pain medication on people who have no pain. Robert F. Cathcart III, currently the physician most experienced in C therapy, found that sick individuals handle extra C differently. They can take much higher oral doses without getting diarrhea. C is most effective when the amount taken is at "bowel tolerance" [when it's on the brink of causing diarrhea]. *If the C intake is not flirting with diarrhea during illness it is not enough and is much less effective.*[5] None of the scientific trials that tested extra C utilized this information.

The timing of C's appearance on the medical scene worked against it also. The advance in technology that led to its being made synthetically led as well to the mass production of "miracle drugs" which revolutionized medical therapy. Penicillin and sulfa had come into general use by 1941. Visions of the future foretold that C could be replaced with prescription drugs. Promotion of it ceased. Treating with it was practically abandoned except in cases of scurvy. This versatile substance, that could rightly be called a miracle drug, ended up in medical limbo alongside healing bracelets and charms worn around the neck.

One can judge that it was more than merely abandoned. It was regarded as a strong competitor that must be discredited regularly in order to prevent its return as the medicine of choice.

The first priority of a pharmaceutical-company scientist is to create a useful drug. The first priority of the marketing division is to win with it in the sales arena, to crowd out all competing products. Hundreds of millions of dollars are at stake. The struggle is war. All is fair. Anything goes. So vitamin C found itself in a war and was ambushed even before its adversary could field a credible army of its own. Yet the generals knew what they were doing. They were looking ahead. They wanted a market to exist for the patentable antiviral drugs they knew they could develop in the future. Until that time the health of the populace---of anyone who was sick---didn't matter. Casualties have always afflicted uninvolved groups during wars. Collateral damage is the current euphemism.

A physician reported in 1938 that injections of C in the form of calcium ascorbate resulted in complete relief or marked improvement in 98 of 100 cases of head colds.[6] Although he attributed most of the benefit to the calcium, word got around that extra C could treat colds. A scientific trial was set up to test the notion. But oral doses were given, not injections. The result, reported in 1942, indicated that C provided no important benefit.[7] The medical community then had scientific evidence that taking C for colds is a useless effort.

Was it a fair trial? *Not at all!* Compare the doses. The total dose used by the physician who injected C averaged 1350 milligrams [mg] per patient. By 1935 it was known that, in order to produce the same benefit, an oral dose of C must be at least *double* the amount given by injection.[8] A comparable oral dose, then, should average 2,700 mg. Some patients would need more, some less. The scientific trial used only 1,000 mg total for each participant. The treatment dose was even less because participants began taking 100 mg of C daily at the start of the cold season, then took an extra 400 mg per day for only two days during a cold. It adds up to 800 mg, less than a third of the 2,700 mg that would equal the average injected amount.

We see that shorting the dose began early in the discrediting of vitamin C.

As young physicians replaced older ones the promise of C faded from the profession's memory. Only a few practitioners were curious enough to continue the evaluation of it in their offices. The benefits they reported lacked the backing of rigorous scientific trials, however. A successful outcome that appeared to be due to extra C may not have been. Before World War II That sort of evidence [termed anecdotal evidence] was acceptable to a degree but afterward times began to change. Any good result from the use of C was either ignored or considered to be due to the nutritive effect on vitamin-deficient patients. Scientific trials that cost millions became the accepted way of proving conclusively that a substance is effective medication. And the physician who neglected to treat with a drug that was approved in this manner became vulnerable to litigation. Physicians who preferred C for a particular malady avoided the threat by treating with both C and an approved drug.

It is mean enough to ignore an excellent therapeutic substance. It is obscene to willfully discredit it. The willful trashing of C by some scientific trials cannot be ruled out. Whenever anecdotal evidence indicated that a diseased condition is treatable with extra C, negative results from one or more scientific trials soon popped up to hammer it back into limbo. While reviewing the medical literature one begins to wonder why anecdotal reports of its effectiveness were always refuted by those trials. Were the good doctors *never* correct? In addition to "proving" that C is ineffective, most reports cautioned that large doses might be toxic---a supremely effective method of conditioning the masses as well as healthcare personnel: Simply provide phony proof that C is worthless plus scare the hell out of them.

Those two ploys account for much of the hesitation to use C in amounts large enough to be effective. Consider the kidney-stone scare. The blanket statement that extra C may cause kidney stones will turn nearly everyone against it. Yet there is no proof by scientific trial that the statement is worthy of consideration. As will be seen in chapter 5 *the evidence indicates that more stones occur in persons who are in the lower range of C consumption!* The stone scare was based mainly on an anecdotal report concerning a few individuals who were prone to develop stones regularly. Physicians who have treated with high-dose C for years state that stones do not occur [chapter 5].

The just-mentioned trial that found C to be of little value in treatment of colds was probably able to influence the healthcare professions so well because many readers of the report lacked the background knowledge necessary for judging it. The report did not refer to the 1938 paper by the physician who treated colds successfully with injected C, therefore no proper dosing schedule was available for comparison. Nor would all readers know that oral doses must be doubled to be as effective as an injected amount.

At that time, anyone who had read both reports would suspect that the 1942 trial was designed to discredit C. And anyone today with adequate background knowledge would generate the same suspicion while reading reports of certain scientific trials conducted during the past 30 years. [This chapter and the three following are involved in supporting that statement.]

In 1996 an editorial in *The Lancet*, a major medical journal, began with this sentence: "Fraud in medical research is prevasive."[9] From the same journal the following year we learn that such misconduct is often condoned, denied or covered up.[10] Fraud is a strong word with startling impact when applied to the conduct of scientists who are supposedly dedicated to improving our health. Fraud does not include rejecting a treatment substance because it is a low-tech nonprescription item, however. *Bias* is the term that applies. It is also pervasive. And although it could very well lead to fraud, it is itself a cause for concern. Let us look into the matter.

You may recall reading a few years ago that scientists at the National Institutes of Health urged volunteers to continue taking an experimental viral hepatitis drug in spite of serious side effects. As a result, five volunteers died, two others survived with liver transplants and several of the luckier ones suffered extensive liver damage.[11] Both the trial and its tragic results were needless. Bias caused the damage. Bias against a low-tech treatment that's been known for years.

In 1954 the AMA journal reported that intravenous infusions of 10 grams of C daily for 5 days were effective against viral hepatitis.[12] In 1960 the *Ohio State Medical Journal* reported that intravenous C cured a case of hepatitis after all other heroic efforts had failed.[13] In 1971 Fred Klenner, the pioneer physician in high-dose C therapy, wrote that his viral-hepatitis patients were well and back to work in 3 to 7 days after treatment with intravenous and oral C.[14] In 1975 Akira Murata, noting that it cuts viral nucleic acid, used C to prevent transfusion hepatitis.[15] In 1981 Robert Cathcart III, mentioned earlier, stated that properly taken *oral* doses will reverse viral hepatitis rapidly.[5,16] Other such reports appear in the medical literature.

So why do we need a toxic high-tech drug for the disease when there are so many reports that C is effective?

Viral hepatitis and shingles are only two of many diseases that can cause severe complications, even death, because of the ingrained bias against the use of vitamin C.

"Hold on," a skeptic would protest, "those so-called cures are only doctor reports, not scientific trials! When the vitamin is tested scientifically it turns out to be no better than dummy pills! It couldn't prevent colds, you know, and didn't stop cancer, so all the doctor reports in the world won't convince me!"

The skeptic stands on solid ground---if the dosing schedules employed successfully by physicians were also used in the trials.

They were not.

Just what *is* a scientific trial? A trial is somewhat scientific if a treatment is compared with other treatments or a placebo such as a dummy pill. Participants who are given the other treatments or the placebo are called *controls.* Assigning participants at random to the control and treatment groups creates a *randomized* trial. This eliminates the use of bias in choosing who gets the treatment under study.

The item in the AMA journal in 1954 [reference 12] about treating hepatitis with C was more than just a doctor's report. It was in the somewhat-scientific category: C was compared with other treatments at the University of Basel and seen to be more effective than the others.

In the more rigorous trials, the individuals under study do not know whether they are taking the treatment being evaluated or are in the *control* group. They're said to be *blinded*. If they are blinded but the scientists are not, it is a *single-blind* trial. If the scientists are also unaware of who is being treated with what, it is a *double-blind* trial.

A randomized, controlled, double-blind trial in which treated groups match the control group with respect to age, sex, ethnic background---and whatever else a critic would find fault with---is the recognized way of learning the truth about a method of treatment. Doctors trust the results obtained by such trials. They may not care to use a treatment that does not have this scientific support. As Dr. Cathcart once remarked, "You know we're all worshipping at the altar of double-blind studies now."[16]

Scientific trials are not designed by deities, however, or conducted by high priests whose only purpose in life is selfless enhancement of the wellbeing of humanity. Before we bow to that altar with unbounded faith we should wonder how all the physicians who have reported that extra C has therapeutic value could have been deluding themselves. Skepticism can cut both ways. Perhaps we'd better see whether the high priests of scientific inquiry have deviated from acceptable ritual and holy purpose. We shall examine closely all the important trials that tested vitamin C.

We'll start with a serious disease that has already been mentioned---viral hepatitis. I just cited some reports that C could treat it. In Tokyo in 1974 a group of microbiologists met in convention to share information. Akira Murata of Japan reported on his studies of bacteriophages---viruses that infect bacteria. He mentioned that earlier scientists had reported C could inactivate both plant and animal viruses---for example, those of herpes, poliomyelitis, rabies, influenza A, cowpox, tobacco mosiac and foot-and-mouth disease.

He said: "...the virucidal activity of C seems to be a phenomenon that is accepted in all viruses." Cutting of the nucleic acid strands is mainly responsible for the inactivation, he added.

A virus injects its DNA into a bacterium which then manufactures more viruses. C degrades viral DNA into lower molecules, thereby preventing proliferation. RNA is degraded in the same manner. Because the damage is limited mostly to viruses suggests that viral nucleic acid is more vulnerable than that of bacteria and other cells.

The second part of Murata's presentation deals with the observations of the chief of surgical services at a hospital where extra C was given to see if it would prevent the viral hepatitis that occurred in about 7% of patients who were given blood transfusions. Benefit appeared to kick in at a dose of 2 grams daily when tried on about 1,100 patients. Similar benefit was seen at another hospital involving about 1,400 patients. A few cases of viral hepatitis did occur, however, but the physicians were not certain that transfusions were the cause.

Because of these questionable cases during the initial observations [not scientific trials] the Japanese physicians began to use daily doses greater than 2 grams in actual hospital practice. Their recommendation: 3 to 6 grams per day in divided doses for a few days before transfusion and for 2 weeks afterward. The C can be given orally or intravenously.

In addition to viral hepatitis, extra C was used for treating mumps; measles; viral orchitis; aphthous stomatitis; shingles; herpes facialis; encephalomyelitis; viral pneumonia and its associated pleuritis; and certain types of meningitis. Murata closed by stating: "The basic and clinical results presented here support the conclusion of L. Pauling, I. Stone and F.R. Klenner that C is effective in both the prevention and treatment of viral diseases." The paper was published by the Science Council of Japan in 1975.[15]

The news that C was recommended for the prevention of viral

hepatitis via transfused blood prompted a group in America to test the advice. The results were reported in the widely read *American Journal of Clinical Nutrition,* January 1981, under this title: VITAMIN C PROPHYLAXIS FOR POSTTRANSFUSION HEPATITIS: LACK OF EFFECT IN A CONTROLLED TRIAL.

Notice that the outcome is revealed in the title. Why should busy doctors read more? All the information they need is transmitted at the beginning of the paper. They would make a mental note that C again failed to live up to its promise and skip the details. Large medical libraries receive more than 3,000 journals relating to healthcare. To keep abreast of so much material not in their special field, doctors scan only titles and abstracts [summaries]. Thus the medical community formed the impression that C cannot prevent transfusion hepatitis.

We shall read beyond the title and abstract. We see that the trial was set up to test Japanese physicians' observation that 2 or more grams of C per day exhibited a preventive effect against transfusion hepatitis. The American trial used an oral dose of 3.2 grams---800 mg given 4 times a day---starting 48 hours before transfusion and continuing for 2 weeks afterward.

Those who would read the report without also reading the one by the Japanese, which was scarce in the U.S., would conclude that an oral dose of 3.2 grams per day was a more-than-adequate test of C as a preventive for transfusion hepatitis. They'd assume that a fair trial had been conducted. *And they'd be conned!* Because **nowhere** in the American report is it mentioned that the Japanese physicians recommended *3 to 6* grams per day! The American dose barely exceeded the minimum!

This is a typical example of the bias against C in the realm of scientific investigation. The trial had not been set up to learn the truth about C. There appears to have been a total lack of holy sincerity on the part of the high-priests who conducted the study. Even so, most members of the healthcare community worshipped at the altar of this double-blind trial.

A proper trial designed to learn the truth should leave no stone unturned. Some participants in such a study should be given the highest dose advised---6 grams intravenously in this case, or 12 grams orally. [You'll recall that, for equal availability to the body, oral C should be twice that given by injection]. The dose range advised allows adjustment for differences in the age, condition and weight of patients. Americans weigh more than Japanese generally, so to assure that no stone be left unturned the American dose should be greater than 6 or 12 grams.

The lack of effect that is claimed in the title is misleading. Of 85 patients on placebo, 8 developed hepatitis. Of 90 on C, 6 developed hepatitis---25% fewer cases in a greater number of participants. If the number of participants are kept below a critical figure, however, it can be said that the difference is not significant, that it may have been by chance. We have no doubt that if a prescription drug had accounted for a 25% reduction in a small trial it would have been followed by a larger one that used higher doses. But just this one small trial was enough to hammer C back into limbo again.

We expect higher ethical behavior in the area of healthcare, a certain gallantry that is not a part of common commerce. We feel that healthcare should be different. We want to trust the system. In contrast, we wouldn't expect a baker to have a moral obligation to tell us that a competitor bakes a better cookie. And suppose he was caught sneaking sand into the better-cookie mix. He'd find himself in court, being ordered to compensate his competitor.

A deceptive scientific trial is the bias-driven equivalent of sneaking sand into rival cookies. Yet in a profession where the result is hazardous to health, when those not swallowing the product whole encounter grit, they merely say the trial is flawed. There is no reckoning. So the deceitful manner in which C is discredited can go on and on without penalty.

The inclination to thwart the therapeutic use of C is not limited to those who design deceptive trials. Medical-journal editors appear biased also. Note this statement in *The Lancet*, July 9, 1994: "Furthermore, although post-transfusion hepatitis B is now considered virtually completely preventable in Japan...." As the commentary continues, *how* the prevention is achieved is never mentioned. *Not a word!* Readers are left to wonder what Japanese physicians do that is not done in other countries.

Experts have warned that future deaths from hepatitis will triple. They called for more research.[17] Are they really blind to the papers on C versus hepatitis referenced here? Or are they just biased? According to the cover story in *U.S. News and World Report*, June 22, 1998, we're going to have to learn to live with hepatitis. The magazine features a "news you can use" section. I sent some of the information in this chapter and offered to send more, at no charge. The editors weren't interested.

One may wonder why there's so much bias against vitamin C but not E or aspirin, which are also nonprescription items. Those two substances are being promoted by the system for a variety of uses in treatment or prevention. Unlike C, however, they are not a serious threat to revenue. C is much more versatile. If doctors would routinely inject it when indicated or if all of the 80% who can tolerate large doses would use it properly the income of the pharmaceutical industry would shrink considerably.

The establishment has tried to bring C under control by prescription but to date has not succeeded. It is tempting to speculate on what would have happened if the vitamin had been patentable and available only by prescription. The populace might have been better served. Large-scale trials would have determined optimum dose schedules for all the ills that C can treat. The severe side effects of certain other drugs would have been avoided. And, after expiration of the patent, C would be as plentiful and inexpensive as it is now, yet its value would have been proven scientifically.

Several years ago, nontoxic, environmentally safe pepper and garlic extracts were found to be good repellents to garden pests. A chemical company was not interested, however, because, a spokesman said, "We're looking for patentable, proprietary products." ...Well, it may be okay to let garden pests dine on plants until something patentable is developed. But it's unconscionable that people must wait and suffer and die because of the bias against unpatentable C.

The late biochemist Irwin Stone had studied C since 1934. His book, *The Healing Factor: Vitamin C Against Disease* (1972, Grosset & Dunlap, New York), is still referred to often. In 1975 he wrote that there's no excuse for anyone dying of a viral disease.[18] Good evidence exists in the medical literature to support the statement but don't count on the proper use of the scientific method to get it carved in granite. Those unnecessary deaths and "flawed" trials demonstrate that there is indeed a bias in medical research which is both hazardous to our health and hostile to the emergence of the truth.

Of all those who knew that C was being treated unfairly by deceptive trials, only Pauling and a few others have blown the whistle.

References

1   Klenner F R.   The treatment of poliomyelitis and other virus diseases with
     Vitamin C.   *Southern Med & Surg*   1949;111:209-14
2   Dainow I.   Note preliminaire sur le traitement de l-herpes et du zona par la
     vitamine C (acide ascorbique).   *Ann Derm Syph*   *1936; 7:817-28*
3   Jungeblut C W.   Further observations on vitamin C therapy in experimental
     poliomyelitis.   *J Experi Med*   1937; 66:459-77
4   Wright I S.   Cevitamic acid (ascorbic acid; crystalline vitamin C); a critical
     analysis of its use in clinical medicine.   *Ann Intern Med*   1938; 12:516-28
5   Cathcart R F.   Vitamin C, titrating to bowel tolerance, anascorbemia, and
     acute induced scurvy.   *Med Hypoth*   1981; 7:1359-76
6   Ruskin S L.   Calcium cevitamate in the treatment of acute rhinitis.
     Ann Otorhinolaryngology   1938; 47:502-11
7   Cowan D H, Diehl H S, Baker A B.   Vitamins for the prevention of colds.
     JAMA   1942; 120:1268-71
8   Hou H C. Comparison of oral and subcutaneous administration of protective
     doses of ascorbic acid (vitamin C).
     Proc Soc Experi Biol Med   1935; 32:1391-2
9   Anon. editorial.   Dealing with deception.   *Lancet*   1996; 347:843
10   Wilmshurst P.   The code of silence.   *Lancet*   1997; 349:567-9
11   News item.   *Wall Street Journal*   May 16, 1994, page B6
12   Baur H, Staub H.   Treatment of hepatitis with infusions of ascorbic acid;
     comparison with other therapies (abstract).   *JAMA*   1954; 156:565
13   Calleja H B, Brooks R H.   Acute hepatitis treated with high doses of
     vitamin C.   *Ohio State Med J*   1960; 56:821-3
14   Klenner F R.   Observations on the dose and administration of ascorbic
     acid when employed beyond the range of a vitamin in human pathology.
     J Applied Nutr   1971; 23:61-88
15   Murata A. Virucidal activity of vitamin C for prevention and treatment of
     viral diseases.   Proceedings of the first intersectional congress of
     IAMS (1974)   *Science Council of Japan*   1975; 3:432-6
16   Luberoff B J.   Symptomectomy with vitamin C. A chat with Robert
     Cathcart, M.D.   *Chemtech*   1978; February: pp76-86
17   *Wall Street Journal*   March 27, 1997, page B9
18   Stone I.   Letter to the editor   *Nutrition Today*   1975; 10:35

2

On Colds: The Anatomy Of A Snow Job

By now most health writers concede that extra C can ease the misery of a cold but remind us regularly there's no proof it can prevent them.   From *Harvard Men's Health Watch*, February 2000: "Although people take vitamin C to prevent infections, the evidence indicates that it is not effective."   From *Better Homes & Gardens*, January 1998: It's a "medical myth" that C can prevent colds.   *Consumer Reports On Health*, November 1998, under the title *C is not for colds* dismissed the pills with 4 words: "They simply don't work."   And added that not one of more than 20 trials found C effective, nor does it speed recovery. In November, 1994 the *Nutrition Action Healthletter* used only 3 words: "It doesn't work."   In *Prevention*, January 1992, a professor of nutrition stated there's little evidence that C can prevent colds; that more studies show it doesn't.   And this comment is seen in the *Tufts University Diet & Nutrition Letter*, July, 1987: "Despite all the claims, extra vitamin C has not been scientifically demonstrated to prevent or cure the common cold---and not because of a lack of trying."

The last part of the statement reeks of bias. It also raises this question: just how *hard* did the researchers try? Had they adjusted the dose to the individual as is done with other medications? Did their trials exclude the 20% who can't take much extra C orally? Did they leave no stone unturned, as should be done in the quest for truth?

If not, we'll feel that we've been conned again by false priests who invited us to worship at a hologram altar. Let's take a good look at the trials, then judge for ourselves whether we were given a definitive answer on C versus colds.

We can't make a proper judgment, however, until we acquire more background knowledge, a credential that many an "expert" has deemed to be quite unnecessary. A lack of familiarity with the subject will expose us to the same trap they have fallen into.

Chapter one's brief account of C in the 1930s is a first step. Next, consider other early observations: Norman Markwell, an Australian, was one of the curious physicians who continued to explore its potential. He wrote of his World War II experience with sick men who were deficient in vitamins A and C. When given the vitamins they recovered as quickly as when given sulfa without the vitamins.

He decided to test C alone for cold prevention, trying first a half gram [500 mg]. As a starting dose it was not enough. After some experimenting he recommended 750 mg or more at the first hint of a cold, the sooner the better, then 500 mg or more 3 or 4 hours later if symptoms persist, the schedule to be continued as needed until symptoms vanish. He stated that no ill effects from extra C occurred.[1] Notice the flexibility in his dose advice: 750 mg *or more*, to be continued *as needed.* There's no limit on the amount or length of treatment. The 750- and 500-mg doses should be considered the recommended minimum.

A Massachusetts physician, Edme Regnier, experimented for 5 years to work out another minimum-dose regimen: 600 or 625 mg at the first symptom of a cold, the sooner the better; 600 mg every 3 hours during the day; 750 at bedtime and 750 on rising; dosing to last 3 or 4 days then tapered off. He advised a 3-hour span between daytime doses because a 4-hour span was not as effective. He referred to the schedule as a "daily dose of 5 grams," and stated that the amount would not prevent all colds but would banish the misery. Unless the schedule is followed scrupulously he felt it better not to take any extra C.[2]

Regnier's observations on the time spans he tried are enlightening. He saw that 400 mg taken every 2 hours were more effective than 800 mg taken every 4 hours. It has long been known that most of an oral dose of C has left the bloodstream within 4 to 6 hours. For greater benefit from extra C, its blood level must be kept high by frequent dosing.

Linus Pauling's book, *Vitamin C and the Common Cold* was first published in 1970 (W.H. Freeman & Co., San Francisco). In chapter 10, on how to control the common cold, he advised a regular daily C intake of 1 or 2 grams. But he stressed individual differences, stating that some persons can remain in good health and free of colds on a quarter of a gram while others may need 5 or more grams a day. He then mentioned dosing with 4 to 10 grams daily when a cold strikes. Two paragraphs later he raised the figures to 10 or 15 grams. The different dose advice reinforces the message that one size does not fit all people.

Pauling was impressed with the results of a double-blind trial reported by Ritzel in 1961.[3] Ritzel wrote of his reason for trying C against colds, referring to the 1954 trial in which C treated viral hepatitis [ref 12 in chapter 1] and to a 1944 study of the effect of various chemicals on an influenza virus. In that study, iodine, formaldehyde, phenol and other strong chemicals quickly inactivated the virus. *And so did vitamin C!* High acidity was not a factor. The researchers wrote: "The pH of the 0.05 N solution of ascorbic acid was between 6 and 7, yet it caused tremendous inactivation from the outset."[4]

Ritzel used a gram a day against a placebo for 5 days with one group and for 7 days with another. He reported that those taking C averaged 39% fewer sick days and 35% fewer symptoms. Pauling stated that the percentages should be 61 and 65. He is correct. Working with the data accompanying the report indicates that either a misprint or a calculating error occurred.

The establishment did not appreciate Pauling's invasion of its turf. Several letters in medical journals deplored his writing a book for the general public instead of presenting his case to the healthcare community. But Pauling knew that evidence pointing to the therapeutic potential of C was being ignored and going public was the only way to get some action. He knew the reason for ignoring the vitamin was financial: a physician's paper showing that C treated colds successfully had been rejected by the editors of 11 different professional journals. One explained that more than 25% of journal ads promote cold remedies or drugs for complications. An article boosting C would chase away advertisers. Some letters to editors asserted that Pauling was out of his area of expertise. The writers may not have known that he had been exploring blood chemistry for years. He was honored in 1963 for unraveling the mystery of sickle cell anemia.

Pauling and his best-seller book could not be dismissed as readily as had other favorable information on C. He had to be agreed with or proven wrong. A rash of scientific trials were set up. Meanwhile, people dosed with C, often improperly, and peppered doctors with dozens of questions about it. Doctors had few answers other than to caution about taking such astronomical amounts.

As for astronomical amounts, Klenner, the pioneer C thera-pist, wrote in 1971 that a gram of C and hour would treat a severe cold [ref 14, chapter 1]. Klenner was not one to fool around with minimum doses. His regimens were so far beyond the ken of the establishment that very few paid any attention.

Regnier's 5-gram daily regimen gathered support in 1973 when a Scottish team reported that a distortion occurs in the white-cell component of the blood soon after a cold strikes.[5] The amount of C in this component drops to about half its normal value for 2 days, then builds back to normal over a period of about 3 more days. To test the value of extra C, participants in a study took a gram a day as a so-called *prophylactic* dose, then 5 more grams when a cold struck---a total daily amount of 6 grams. Dosing remained at this level for at least 3 days before reverting to the continuous gram a day.

That regimen prevented the distortion---*and the cold also!*

In conclusion, the Scottish researchers advised taking from 6 to 10 grams of C a day when a cold threatens.

[The drop in C that occurs in the white-cell component was explained several years later: Usually, white-cell C is measured in the so-called buffy layer of centrifuged blood. The layer includes all types of white cell as well as platelets. One type of white cell, the monocyte, contains more than twice the amount of C that is found in other types. When a cold strikes, large numbers of low-C white cells move into the bloodstream, thus diluting the C content of a thimbleful of buffy-layer fluid. It's like diluting an elite well-armed division with thousands of poorly-armed recruits. Fighting efficiency drops. Taking extra C provides the "firepower" that restores the combat readiness of the body. Stresses other than colds also distort the white-cell picture. Distortion occurs after a heart attack, for example, and lingers for more than 4 months.[6]]

Looking back, we see that Regnier, the Massachusetts physician, eliminated the misery of colds with 5 grams of C a day. His participants did not take a daily prophylactic gram. They took extra C only after a cold threatened. Those in the Scottish study, however, took a daily gram of C even when colds were not coming on. They raised their intake by 5 grams, to 6 per day, when a cold threatened. They could not suppress the cold with only a 4-gram rise. So we see that 5 grams a day suppressed colds in the Massachusetts study but in the Scottish study, 1 gram plus 4 more did not.

What does that tell us? *It tells us that a **continuous** dose of C is of little value in cold treatment!* The 5-gram *rise* in dose can't be reduced by any amount taken continuously. This effect, a tolerance to extra C, has been seen in other studies also. Realizing that it occurs is very important to the understanding of how to take C properly. In the minimum dose range, we can't be taking, say, 3 grams a day and expect to suppress a cold by adding another 3 grams. Even adding 6 grams may not be enough. The more C taken continuously, the more **additional** C required to overcome the tolerance effect.

I imagine it's a concept every wino is familiar with.

Now we have enough background knowledge to judge the trials that pitted C against the common cold. We will examine the ones reported in the 1970s and 1980s that were started after Pauling's book came out in 1970. Most of them were started after the Scottish team found a 5-gram *rise* in the daily dose is necessary---and that it must be kept high for at least 3 days.

A fair trial should test the regimens that physicians had reported to be effective. To leave no stone unturned, some should have used Klenner's gram-an-hour schedule. But we won't be so demanding. All we wish to see are the results of a trial which, at the first symptom of a cold, used a 5-gram *rise*, kept that high for at least 3 days. Or one in which the doses were taken every 3 hours or less during the daytime. Or one that employed Markwell's *or more* and *as needed* adjustment. Or any combination of the above. Those are the recommendations of practicing physicians, not Pauling.

In a sense, Pauling should be thought of as the *messenger* who distributed the information that physicians had gathered during treatments. But he was more than that. He salted in his own observations, opinions and personal experience. He used his reputation as a brilliant scientist to rock the boat. It threatened the economic way of life in certain circles.

The reaction was to kill the messenger.

Two nutritionists launched an early attack on him with an unfavorable review of his book in the *Canadian Medical Association Journal*, August 21, 1971. They deplored his spreading of untested theories, noting that disparaging remarks by other reviewers included the term "near quackery." Pauling replied that Ritzel's trial was a good enough test---and that even the low dose used in a 1942 trial [ref 7, chapter 1] demonstrated that C was of *some* value. He then wrote that about 200 mg of C a day would result in 15% fewer colds; and a continuous gram a day would reduce the incidence of colds by 45% and total illness by 60% [*Canadian Medical Association Journal*, Sept 4, 1971].

By relying on Ritzel's one-week trial on boys aged 15 to 17 years and overlooking the tolerance effect, Pauling moved far out on a limb. If he meant to goad critics into setting up trials, he succeeded. Scores of them sharpened their saws. Incidentally, Ritzel's report did not state the age or sex of the participants in his study. The information appears in Pauling's 1976 book, *Vitamin C and the Common Cold and the Flu* [W.H. Freeman & Co., San Francisco].

Our look at the trials begins with Anderson's. His group's first trial, reported in 1972, used 4 grams---a continuous dose of a gram a day which was raised by 3 grams when a cold occurred. The 3-month-long double-blind study in the Toronto area was done well on cold-prone adults, average age about 29 years. He stated that he added the 3-gram rise in dose when a cold occurred in order to follow Pauling's recommendation. Remember, however, that Pauling's advice ranged from 4 to 15 grams per day. Testing only the minimum dose, which is below that shown to be adequate by physicians, leaves a lot of stones unturned.

Although the study failed to use higher doses, the results were impressive. Significantly more individuals in the C group remained free of illness. *Isn't that scientific proof that a number of colds were prevented?* The duration of colds in those who did get them was shorter by 21% in the C group; and total illness was reduced by 30%. But Anderson was not inclined to join Pauling out on the limb. He felt that no firm recommendation could be made at the time regarding the use of extra C.[7]

The Anderson group's second 3-month-long double-blind study, reported in 1974, was designed to determine whether the value of C was due to the gram-a-day continuous dose, the 3 grams added when a cold struck, or both. The combination was slightly more effective. Several other regimens were tested also.

Little benefit resulted from continuous doses of a fourth gram, 1 gram and 2 grams. The smallest amount performed as well as the largest. Anderson surmised that the participants, all adults, were well enough nourished so that added C did not increase their resistance to illness.

The study's important finding emerged from the two higher doses tested: Participants who took 8 grams on the first day of a cold, but no more later, had less illness than those who took 4 grams in that manner. He noted that the result agreed with the finding of the Scottish team---that higher doses may be required for the suppression of colds in most individuals.[8]

But in his final study, a 15-week double-blind effort reported in 1975, Anderson showed no interest in confirming that higher doses might prevent nearly all colds. In this trial, a half gram of C was taken once a week for the duration. Apart from the weekly half gram, 1.5 grams were taken on the first day of a cold, then the dose was reduced to 1 gram daily for the next 4 days. Timed-release pills were slightly more effective than standard ones. Participants who took C spent about 25% less time indoors due to illness than did those on placebo.

The impressive figure prompted Anderson to state: "Taken in conjunction with the positive results reported by other investigators, there is now little doubt that intake of additional vitamin C can lead to a reduced burden of winter illness." But he concluded by stating there's an upper limit to "useful regular supplementation" with C and that higher doses risk the possibility of toxic effects and dependency.[9]

The mention of toxicity is warranted because rare sensitivities, not only with respect to C but to *every* substance, are lurking in the human gene pool. The side effects of aspirin and other drugs are more dangerous but warnings about them are not as numerous. Perhaps the toxicity word was included in so many reports on C in the 1970s because much of the knowledge of the 1930s had been forgotten. Or was it to add more weight to the hammer that would pound the vitamin into limbo again?

Dependency is discussed in chapter 5. Comment here is limited to noting that it will not occur when using high-dose C to abort a cold then tapering off in a few days.

Chronological order was disregarded by looking first at Anderson's 3 trials. A report by Charleston and Clegg preceded Anderson's 1972 report by 3 months. In this single-blind study 47 adults in Glasgow took a continuous [prophylactic] gram of C per day after breakfast, with no increase during colds. Of that group, 16 had no cold during the 16-week trial period. Only 6 of 43 on placebo had no cold. The 31 on C who did get colds had a total of 44 while the 37 in the placebo group logged 80.[10]

In 1973 Schwartz reported a double-blind study on 21 cold-susceptible male prisoners who were additionally confined to hospital for 4 weeks. After a week of observation, 11 took a gram of C a day for 3 weeks while 10 took placebo in the same manner. When they had taken the pills for 2 weeks, a half milliliter of fluid containing a cold virus was dripped into each nostril. All developed colds in 12 to 24 hours. Except for one man, colds in the C group began to clear up sooner than in those on placebo. Except for quicker recovery, C was of limited value.[11] Although the conditions would not occur normally, the study shows that 3 grams, subject to the tolerance effect for 2 weeks, cannot inactivate a substantial viral inoculation.

Elliott reported a 10-week double-blind study in 1973 on confined males also---70 of the 140 sailors aboard a Polaris submarine at a time when they exposed each other to viruses acquired while on their simultaneous leave. The men endure an epidemic of new colds every time they get together again for duty. On half-gram doses taken 4 times a day, 37 on C had as many runny noses and sneezes as 33 on placebo but were not as sick by an average of 34%.[12]

Carson reported 2 double-blind 80-day studies in 1974 via a letter to the editor of the *British Medical Journal* rather than the usual long paper with charts and statistical crunch-outs. A continuous gram of C per day was used in both trials, in one as a single effervescent drink and in the other as a half-gram pill taken twice daily. The study, on adults in southern England, focused only the number of colds. No difference was seen between the 153 on C and 142 on placebo.[13]

Coulehan reported a 14-week double-blind C trial on Navaho children in 1974. Those aged 6 to 10 years took a single-dose gram a day while those aged 10 to 15 years took a single-dose 2 grams daily. The 321 on C and 320 on placebo had the same number of colds but sick days were fewer by 34% in those on 2 grams of C and 28% fewer in children taking 1 gram. In concluding, Coulehan wrote: "...there are enough data suggesting a beneficial influence of vitamin C on respiratory infections to warrant further investigations."[14]

We depart from chronological order again to review the 1976 double-blind trial report by Coulehan. 428 Navaho children, ages 6 through 15, took a gram of C a day. [Note that it was half the earlier dose taken by the older children.] A matched number took placebo. The meals of both groups contained more C than the RDA, suggesting that they were well nourished. No real difference in illness was seen, except that 13 on placebo had positive beta-hemolytic strep cultures, versus 6 in the C group. Coulehan concluded: "...we do not believe that vitamin C has widespread usefulness as a cold remedy." A footnote in the report states that the opinions expressed in the paper do not necessarily reflect the views of the Indian Health Service.[15]

Coulehan later reviewed the studies of C versus colds done prior to 1978 and found "no reason to accept Pauling's contention" that large doses of C can prevent or cure acute or chronic illness other than scurvy.[16] David Bee, a California physician, responded by pointing out the one element biased persons omit: the trials did not test Pauling's entire dose range. Bee wrote that on many patients, as well as himself, "...3 to 4 gm up to 6 times a day for a total daily dose of 10 to 15 gm are necessary to obtain relief of cold symptoms." And : "It puzzles me that the studies done to test Pauling's hypothesis have not actually followed his recommendations." In reply, Coulehan pointed to Anderson's use of 8 grams of C.[17] But Coulehan did not mention that the dose was taken for one day only, or that it was more effective than 4 grams taken for one day only. Pauling's recommendation of 10 to15 grams "per day" on page 86 of his 1970 book does not imply that dosing be limited to one day only.

Briggs, in a 1974 report of an ongoing double-blind C study, wrote that 50 mg taken daily and raised to 200 mg at the start of a cold was as effective as a gram daily that was raised to 4 grams when a cold occurred.[18] The study went on through 8 Australian winters. Final results, not differing from the 1974 report, were published in a book he edited [*Recent Vitamin Research*, 1984, CRC Press, Boca Raton, Florida]. There was no placebo group. The 50-mg daily dose taken by one group assured that all participants had enough C so that study results would not be skewed in favor of C by the malnutrition factor.

In 1974 Sabiston and Radomski reported on 2 groups of Canadian soldiers conducting a military exercise in the far north. Of the 56 men who took a half gram of C twice daily, 6 colds occurred, versus 14 in the same number who took placebo. In many men the blood level of C was low at the start. Their rations supplied only about 40 mg a day, mostly in a drink that was often discarded. Duration of colds was the same in both groups but those on C had milder symptoms.[19] There is no mention that the study was double-blind.

In 1975 Clegg and Macdonald reported a double-blind 15-week study on 3 groups of university students in Glasgow. A group of 67 took a gram of C a day, 70 took placebo and 74 took D-isoascorbic acid, a man-made isomer of C that is also called erythorbic acid. Little difference in number of colds was seen in the C and placebo groups but those who took D-isoascorbic acid had 34% fewer colds than the other groups.[20] No other long study of this "false" C versus colds is in the literature. Its ability to prevent scurvy is nearly zero but, like C, it is virucidal.

In 1975 Karlowski reported a 9-month trial, said to be double-blind, in which 6 grams of C were taken for 5 days.[21] Readers might think that a trial using adequate doses had at last been conducted. But those who know C well would suspect that a clever arrangement of the dosing schedule had occurred. Done in the Washington, D.C. area on 190 total subjects, the trial was "rushed into operation" so that "There was no time to design, test, and have manufactured a placebo that would be indistinguishable from ascorbic acid." [Quotes are in the report.]

One may wonder why the hurry and why funding was granted so quickly. The answer may be that in March, 1973 news of the Scottish study that 6 grams of C a day could prevent colds called for a quick application of spin control, a Washington specialty, to counter the notion that higher doses of C really can prevent colds. So the rush was on to get a trial underway by fall.

As in the Scottish study, 6 grams of C a day were used. The Scots reported positive results from a 5-gram *rise* that was added to a 1-gram continuous dose. The Karlowski group reported negative results from a 3-gram *rise* added to a 3-gram daily intake that had been started in September, allowing ample time for tolerance to develop in the C group before the cold season. And when colds did occur the participants had to report for a check of signs and symptoms before they were given extra pills. The delay of up to 24 hours allowed the disease to become well established and more difficult to suppress.

Colds and fires have some features in common, one being that they cannot be doused with the small amount of douser that would have doused earlier. Much more than a minimum dose is needed to suppress an established cold. We might suspect that the researchers were aware of this, for they justified the delay by citing a 1968 study that found taking C at the first sign of a cold to be of no significance. That study used only 3 grams of C however. It teaches nothing more than to reinforce the fact that an inadequate dose is a mere nuisance to a cold virus. Klenner's gram-an-hour regimen, or even more C, is necessary after a cold has progressed beyond the first symptoms. By then the dosing is not for prevention but for avoidance of misery, complications and downtime.

In 1976 Elwood reported a 100-day study in South Wales on women only. The C group, 339, took a gram a day while 349 took placebo. He saw a "small preventive effect" on chest colds in the C group. Whether it was blinded is not mentioned.[22]

Elwood reported another trial, double-blind, in 1977, also in South Wales, which included the women's husbands, roughly 525 couples. Husband and wife received the same type of 1-gram pill, either C or placebo. Each was given 10 and told to take 3 a day on the first 3 days of a cold and 1 on the fourth day. Elwood concluded that the effect of C on the common cold "is at best elusive and probably trivial."[23] This is to be expected when colds last longer than the supply of C.

Tyrrell's double-blind study on 1524 adults in the London, England area, reported in 1977, allowed C to run out in mid-cold also. Each person was given 10 pills, either C or placebo, and told to take 4 of them a day when a cold came on. The poor results from a regimen that lasted just 2.5 days provided no reason for him to recommend C for colds.[24]

In 1977 Ludvigsson reported 2 double-blind trials conducted in Sweden. The first, a 7-week study in spring with 158 children, age 8 or 9; the second, of 3-months duration in fall with 615 children, also 8 or 9 years of age. Roughly half in each trial took a gram of C a day. So that low dietary C would not be a factor, the placebo contained a little C, 30 mg in spring and 10 mg in fall. Colds were about equal in both well-nourished groups.[25]

Miller reported a 5-month double-blind Indiana trial in 1977 that used identical twins, aged 6 to 15 years. One of each pair took C, 500, 750 or 1,000 mg, depending on weight. Although the meager amounts provided some benefit it was not significant. But in 6 of the 7 youngest pair of boys the twin who took a half gram of C grew taller than his brother by an average of 1.3 centimeters. One grew 2.54 centimeters, a full inch taller.[26]

For 8 weeks Pitt and Costrini gave 331 Marine recruits a gram of C each morning and night while 343 took placebo during a double-blind study reported in 1979. Colds were about equal in both groups but questionnaire data indicated they were less severe in the C group, which also had only 1 of 8 pneumonia cases. The C group logged more sick calls and training days lost to colds, however. One man on C was removed from the study after he developed a rash whenever extra C was taken.[27]

In 1981 Carr reported a 100-day double-blind study in which one adult took a gram of C a day while his or her identical twin took placebo during winter in Sydney, Australia. In number, colds were about equal but shorter by 19% in the C group.[28]

In Coronel during a Chilean winter Bancalari's double-blind 12-week study, reported in 1984, had 32 children aged 10 to 12 years take 2 grams of C a day while 30 took placebo. Result: 37% less illness in the C group, which also had slightly fewer colds and recovered a day sooner than did those on placebo.[29]

The list of cold trials ends with Mink's double-blind study reported in 1988. By using men who were vulnerable to a specific virus his Wisconsin team reduced certain variables that tended to distort the results of many studies. Serum C was measured at the start and seen to be about equal in the C and placebo groups. The 2 groups then started taking their pills---500 mg 4 times a day. After 3.5 weeks the serum and white-cell C content was measured and the men were housed for a week with 8 men who had been given colds from a single virus. During that time and for 2 weeks afterward the C and placebo groups continued to take their pills. Colds were caught by 4 of the 8 men in the C group and by 7 of the 8 taking placebo. Signs and symptoms in the placebo group were much more severe.[30]

After reading these reports, only stubborn bias would induce a person to still insist that C---even as little as a gram or two a day---cannot prevent colds in some persons and reduce illness in many more. And only bias would prompt a person to insist that the trial doses equaled those used successfully by physicians.

A summary of the cold studies. Many used more than one dose size but to avoid clutter only the highest is listed. Dosing days are shown only if the daily dose reached 5 grams, the minimum advised by Regnier. Under **GRAMS**, the number in parentheses is the amount of C taken daily prior to a **rise** when a cold occurred. It is of little value in cold treatment. Only Anderson, Karlowski and Briggs used a continuous dose that was increased during colds.

YEAR	LEAD AUTHOR (S)	GRAMS
1972	Anderson	3 (1)
	Charleston, Clegg	1
1973	Elliott	2
	Schwartz	3
1974	Carson	1
	Coulehan	2
	Briggs	3 (1)
	Sabiston, Radomski	1
	Anderson, for 1 day	8
1975	Anderson	1.5
	Clegg, Macdonald	1
	Karlowski, for 5 days	3 (3)
1976	Elwood	1
	Coulehan	1
1977	Ludvigsson	1
	Miller	1
	Elwood	3
	Tyrrell	4
1979	Pitt, Costrini	2
1981	Carr	1
1984	Bancalari	2
	Briggs (ongoing from '74)	3 (1)
1988	Mink	2

Notice that *no trial* maintained a 5-gram *rise* in dose for at least 3 days.   Many plowed the same ground that had been worked before, with doses low enough to guarantee failure [and assure publication].   The flow of negative results from trial after trial bombarded the public with the regularity of a commercial.

After the first few trial results were published Pauling could see the trend toward discrediting him and published a second book, mentioned earlier, about colds and flu in which he advised as much as 20 grams a day for colds and a gram an hour for flu.

He blasted *Consumer Reports* for its "thoroughly biased report, consisting almost entirely of false statements and seriously misleading statements." [*Consumer Reports* is a fine magazine but it does appear that its editors were, and still are, misled by medical advisers.]   He was frustrated by the devious attitude of the healthcare establishment and a brush-off by the FDA.   The Nobel Laureate had marched into the valley of reputational death while cannon to the right of him, left of him and in front of him volley'd and thunder'd.   He emerged to fight again but the negative results emphasized by media people not knowledgeable enough to have gained perspective, plus disparagement by the 20% who can't take enough C to subdue viruses, undercut his hope of ending the misery of winter illness.

Taken as a group, the cold-trial results we put our trust in add up to a shabby snow job.   We trusted the system to look after our stake in the matter and the system betrayed our trust.   *We're being shafted!*.   Shafted in an area where it hurts the most---our health.   The health of our families, from children with severe viral illness to adults and oldsters with viral hepatitis or shingles or other viral diseases.   Members of the establishment appear determined to prevent publication of an objective study that would prove the antiviral nature of C.

Shafted for what reason?   Money, of course.   There's just too much money at stake to allow high-dose C its rightful place in medical therapy as a versatile antitoxic and antiviral substance.

The system will let you die before it will allow C to shrink the market for proprietary pharmaceuticals.

Who's to blame for this sorry state? Certainly not our doctors. They've been deceived along with the rest of us. They haven't time to do all the reading on this one subject that is needed to assess the validity of the trials. They expect the designers of those trials to be worthy of trust. Blame human nature, I guess. None of us wants to lose income. We want *more*. Nearly everyone in the system gets *more* by sweeping C under the rug.

To spell it out, researchers want to be published. Papers showing that C fails to provide therapeutic benefits are more apt to be accepted. Editors want advertising revenue. And advertisers detest competing products.

Medical journals may be advertising vehicles first and medical journals second. Publishing companies own many of them. The conflict of interest should be obvious. Other journals are owned by the various medical organizations. Their editors, who may not be physicians, in addition to pleasing advertisers, tend to reject papers that would lower the income of organization members. Cathcart stated that his papers on the therapeutic use of C were "flat-out refused." [ref 16, chapter 1.] The fact that much of his important information on C appeared in a chemical-industry journal instead of a major medical journal where it belongs demonstrates how difficult it is to present the truth to members of the healthcare professions.

Some of the best information on C was published by journals that have limited readership and carry few ads---the reason several have ceased publication. One would think that praising C is an ad-dependent publication's way of committing suicide. Note: The January, 1999 issue of *American Health*, instead of recommending the usual few-hundred milligrams of C for treating a cold, advised taking 4,000 mg 3 times a day---12 grams of power! The magazine ceased publication shortly afterward.

[Perhaps it was in terminal agony before then and the editors, having nothing to lose, decided to give C a break for a change.]

Journal editors are gatekeepers. They do not close the gate completely against C. A few reports of favorable anecdotal evidence and results of small trials may squeeze through, as well as studies on the molecular level. But you can bet the home that a proper large-scale scientific trial of C versus a virus, with enough participants to provide statistically powerful data, will never be published. Therefore it will never be funded.

C.W.M. Wilson, a recognized Dublin authority on C, in answer to a query about its safety sent to him by a journal in 1975, slipped in advice for treating colds: 2 grams taken 4 times a day.[31] He may have done more blood studies on C than anyone else. Prior to 1970 he had tried lower doses for colds. One would expect to see a post-Pauling trial by him but he probably decided not to enter that circus because a report that proved C to be quite effective would not have been published anyway.

A company that makes or markets C couldn't recover the cost of a large-scale study. Besides, the company probably would have more profitable products that compete with C. Government grants have funded some C studies but I'm not aware of money for clinical trials that has reached unbiased groups. A few years ago I wrote to the Office of Alternative Medicine, hoping that someone there would see the need for proper clinical trials. Nothing came of it. Any action would have rocked the boat.

Researchers must adapt to that fact of life. An item in *Science*, October 18, 1991, quoted a scientist who deplored the bias against C but didn't care to be identified. Another with similar feelings was concerned about being labeled a C booster. Career advancement might suffer. And a third felt embarrassed and "very awkward" while presenting evidence favorable to C to a skeptical audience. Scientists who study C were said to be like commedian Rodney Dangerfield, who always complained that he got no respect. Work in an atmosphere of that sort is bound to result in wasted grants for flawed trials.

Virologists have a serious conflict of interest in regard to C. They're busy developing their own antiviral drugs. Don't expect *them* to praise the competition. They're more likely to exhibit alarm and utter *"Toxic!"* if someone should mention the vitamin. This from a group whose creations are notoriously toxic! You'll recall that 5 volunteers died after taking one of their drugs for viral hepatitis [page 7].

We should realize by now that, due to individual differences, a gram or two of C may or may not prevent a cold or reduce its misery. In some persons an inadequate dose may even be detrimental. Regnier wrote that he once kept a cold active for about 27 days, "...alternately suppressing it and permitting it to recur by altering the amount of ascorbic acid I took." Each time the cold came on again it was more difficult to suppress until finally he used penicillin to treat the accompanying bacterial infection. He had mentioned a history of respiratory and ear complications that suggested a weak immune response.

Klenner, the pioneer in C therapy, found that doses must not only be adequate but given until the last sign and symptom of illness has vanished. He treated his 7-year-old son's flu-like symptoms with sporadic doses of C, 5 to 10 grams orally, plus a sulfa drug. Treatment was suspended when the condition improved. Three times the disease recurred and was suppressed in that manner. The fourth time it flared up during the 6-week period the treatment was useless. Klenner wrote: "On the third day of this illness the child suddenly became lethargic and just as suddenly to frank stupor. The temperature which had been running low grade was now 102.6. At this point all oral medication was discontinued. I immediately gave 6 grams of ascorbic acid intravenously with a 30 cc syringe. He was awake and asking 'what happened' in 5 minutes."

The boy received another 6-gram IV dose 4 hours later and 2 more 6 hours apart. He was well in 24 hours but 5 grams of C were given orally "in juice" every 8 hours for a week. Then the boy was put back on his usual 7 grams a day. [That's not a misprint. Klenner gave each of his 3 children a gram of C a day for each year the child was old until age ten. Thereafter the dose remained at 10 grams a day unless illness required more.]

The children's doses are good to remember whenever a friend gasps as you pop a couple of gram tablets after lunch. Your friend might also gasp if you'd mention Pauling's latest dose advice. The *Pauling Institute Newsletter* of winter 1992-3 advises 1 or 2 grams of C at the first hint of a cold, then a gram or two every half hour or hour until symptoms vanish. At maximum it exceeds Klenner's gram-an-hour regimen and Irwin Stone's half teaspoon of ascorbate [which has slightly less C] every half hour. Stone wrote that about 95% of colds would vanish by the third or fourth dose [ref 18, chapter 1]. Unless the virus is especially vicious, the total intake for the average cold would be about 16 grams. Cathcart calls the more severe ones "100-gram colds" and treats with that amount daily.

There are good reasons for treating a cold with more than a minimum dose. Eliminating the virus as soon as possible avoids complications that cause a cold to drag on and on. The "cold" actually may be mistaken for flu, which requires much higher doses. Extra C can battle whatever is attacking while helping with the diagnosis. If much more C is needed to banish ache-all-over symptoms, suspect flu. Still another reason for tak- more than a minimum amount is that our C intake is higher than it used to be. Because of the tolerance effect, this increased intake appears to render inadequate the doses that had been effective earlier. You'll recall that IV doses averaging 1,350 mg gave complete relief from head colds in 1938 [page 5].

The tolerance effect may also kick in because of the sodium erythorbate in our food. It is a salt of erythorbic acid that Clegg and Macdonald tested against colds [page 26]. This virtual twin of C is often used instead of C to improve certain foods, such as canned applesauce and pie fillings. The package labels of bacon, hot dogs and other processed meat list as an ingredient either sodium erythorbate ["false C"] or true C. One or the other is added to reduce cancer-causing nitrosamines that form when the meat is cooked. In 1996 it was estimated that more than 200 mg of erythorbate per capita is added to our food supply every day, close to 3 times the new RDA for true C.[32] This man-made substance may be still another reason why we now need more C to reduce the misery of colds.

One can feel a bit uneasy about getting so much false C in our food every day. Erythorbate is not allowed in European food. Its antiscurvy power is near zero. What other important function does it lack? In many respects the body assumes it is true C. It shows up as C in blood and urine tests unless an improved method is used [HPLC]. Although much of it is destroyed in cooking, people who consume several ounces of luncheon meat or other cold foods laced with it may be ingesting more false C than true C. Erythorbate is said to be harmless---but so were certain food dyes and hydrogenated oils.

The 1996 study suggests that erythorbate neither helps nor hinders the action of true C, even though erythorbate concentration in certain white cells [monocytes] can be up to 40% of true C present. The effect in sickness is not known, as the study was done on healthy young women.[32] In the old and sick, 40% of the molecules doing nothing might interfere with the action of true C. Since years may pass before a pattern is perceived, let's hope that a harmful feature of sodium erythorbate is not a part of our future. I avoid products that contain it.

We have arrived at the end of this chapter with a better understanding of C. Some questions may have arisen, such as: If we prevent all colds for a time, then could get no more C, would the next cold be quite severe? Probably; our antibody memories might be too dim to respond quickly. For some, it might be better to keep C in reserve and use it only when a cold threatens to disrupt a major event in their lives. It seems that people should be curious enough to learn whether they can tolerate large doses. And if so, to prove for themselves that proper doses *can* prevent colds. The establishment will never do it.

Chapter 2 References

1   Markwell N W. Vitamin C in the prevention of colds.
     Med J Australia 1947; 2:777-8

2   Regnier E. The administration of large doses of ascorbic acid in the
     prevention and treatment of colds (part 2).
     Review of Allergy 1968; 22:948-56

3   Ritzel Von G. Kritische Beurteilung des Vitamins C als Prophylacticum
     Therapeuticum der Erkaltungskrankheiten.
     Helvetia Medica Acta 1961; 1:63-8

4   Knight C A, Stanley W M. The effect of some chemicals on purified
     influenza virus. *J Experimental Med* 1944; 209:291-300

5   Hume R, Weyers E. Changes in leucocyte ascorbic acid during the
     common cold. *Scot Med J* 1973; 18:3-7

6   Vallance B D, Hume R, Weyers E. Reassessment of changes in
     leucocyte and serum ascorbic acid after acute myocardial infarction.
     Brit Heart J 1978; 40:64-8

7   Anderson T W, Reid D B W, Beaton G H. Vitamin C and the common
     cold; a double-blind trial. *Can Med A J* 1972; 107:503-8

8   Anderson T W, Suranyi G, Beaton G H. The effect on winter illness of
     large doses of vitamin C. *Can Med A J* 1974; 111:31-6

9   Anderson T W, Beaton G H, Corey P N, Spero L. Winter illness and
     vitamin C; the effect of relatively low doses.
     Can Med A J 1975; 112:823-6

10   Charleston S S, Clegg K M. Ascorbic acid and the common cold.
     Lancet 1972; 1:1401-2

11   Schwartz A R, Togo Y, Hornick R B, et al. Evaluation of the efficacy of
     ascorbic acid in prophylaxis of induced rhinovirus 44 infection in man.
     J Infect Dis 1973; 128:500-5

12   Elliott B. Ascorbic acid: efficacy in the prevention of symptoms of
     respiratory infection on a Polaris submarine.
     Internat'l Research Communications Sys. Med Science 1973; 1(3):12

13   Carson M, Corbett M, Cox H, Pollitt N. Vitamin C and the common cold
     Brit Med J 1974; March 23 p 577

14   Coulehan J L, Reisinger K S, Rogers K D, Bradley D W.
     Vitamin C prophylaxis in a boarding school. *N Engl J Med* 1974; 200:6-10

15   Coulehan J L, Eberhard S, Kapner L, et al. Vitamin C and acute illness in
     Navajo schoolchildren. *N Engl J Med* 1976; 295:973-7

16   Coulehan J L. Ascorbic acid and the common cold: reviewing the evidence.
     Postgrad Med 1979; 66:153-60

17   Bee D M, (letter) and Coulehan J L. (letter) The vitamin C controversy.
     Postgrad Med 1980; 67:64 and 69

18   Briggs M H. Clinical trials with vitamin C. *Lancet* 1974; 2:1211-12

19   Sabiston B H, Radomski M W. Health problems and vitamin C in Canadian
     northern military operations. DCIEM Biosci Div Report 74-R-1012, March
     1974 Defence Research Board--Dept Nat'l Defence--Canada.

38

Chapter 2 References

20 Clegg K M, Macdonald J M. L-ascorbic acid and D-isoascorbic acid in a common cold survey. *Am J Clin Nutr* 1975; 28:973-6

21 Karlowski I R, Chalmers T C, Frankel L D, et al. Ascorbic acid for the common cold; a prophylactic and therapeutic trial. *JAMA* 1975; 231:1038-42

22 Elwood P C, Lee H P, St. Leger A S, et al. A randomized controlled trial of vitamin C in the prevention and amelioration of the common cold. *Brit J Prev Soc Med* 1976; 30:193:6

23 Elwood P C, Hughes S J, St. Leger A S. A randomized controlled trial of the therapeutic effect of vitamin C in the common cold. *Practitioner* 1977; 218:133-7

24 Tyrrell D A J, Craig J W, Meade T W, White T. A trial of ascorbic acid in the treatment of the common cold. *Brit J Prev Soc Med* 1977; 31:189-91

25 Ludvigsson J, Hansson L O, Tibbling G. Vitamin C as a preventive medicine against common colds in children. *Scand J Infec Dis* 1977; 9:91-8

26 Miller J Z, Nance W E, Norton J A, et al. Therapeutic effect of vitamin C; a co-twin control study. *JAMA* 1977; 237:248-51

27 Pitt H A, Costrini A M. Vitamin C prophylaxis in Marine recruits. *JAMA* 1979; 241:908-11

28 Carr A B, Einstein R, Lai L Y C, et al. Vitamin C and the common cold; using identical twins as controls. *Med J Australia* 1981; 2:411-12

29 Bancalari A, Seguel C, Neira F, et al. Prophylactic value of vitamin C in acute respiratory infections of schoolchildren. *Rev Med Chili* 1984; 112:871-6

30 Mink K A, Dick E C, Jennings L C, Inhorn S L. Amelioration of rhinovirus colds by vitamin C (ascorbic acid) supplementation. *Med Virology VII*, 1988:356. In De La Maza L M, Peterson E M, Eds. *Proc International Symposium on Medical Virology*; Elsevier Press, Amsterdam, 1988

31 Wilson C W M. Ascorbic acid and the common cold. *Practitioner* 1975; 215:343-5

32 Sauberlich H E, Tamura T, Craig C B, et al. Effects of erythorbic acid in vitamin C metabolism in young women. *Am J Clin Nutr* 1996; 64:336-46

3

On Cancer: Deceptive Clinical trials

In chapter 1, an inadequate dose and a small number of participants were used to demonstrate scientifically that C could not treat viral hepatitis. And although the C group had 25% fewer cases of the disease, the small number of participants allowed the claim that the result may have occurred by chance.

In chapter 2, inadequate doses; delay of the first one; long time spans between them; curtailing days of treatment; and the tolerance effect were used to discredit C as a preventive or treatment of the common cold.

In this third chapter we examine the trials with C versus cancer. Did clever trial design serve to discredit C in this area also? Before we can answer correctly, we must again acquire background knowledge and read entire trial reports, not just titles and abstracts.

C has been shown to inactivate cancer cells in a test tube. The authors of the report stated that nontoxic substances "have been largely if not totally excluded from consideration" by a national cancer center looking for new treatments.[1] For a long time conventional wisdom held that cancer drugs must be toxic. Not so now. More and more benign substances are showing promise, such as one in human milk[2] and a drug for treating chronic myelogenous leukemia, trademarked Gleevec,[3] that works well for a time in some individuals.[4] It has been seen to shrink a type of gastrointestinal tumor and is being tried on other cancers.[5]

All sorts of treatment have been tried for cancer. The unconventional ones are usually touted by quacks more concerned with income than benefit to patients. But reputable physicians with commendable motives have also tried unconventional therapy.

In the journal *Cancer Surveys* [1989; 8:713-23], Helen Nauts wrote an absorbing account of cancer regression due to purulent bacterial infection followed by fever. The infection must be of bacterial origin, not viral. She wrote: "...the largest number of permanent cures followed the more prolonged infections, principally staphylococcal." Erysipelas, a streptococcal infection, was the most effective in regressing advanced cancer, however.

Nauts referred to a case that was reported before 1744. it concerned a woman with breast cancer that had advanced to the hopeless stage. She developed an abscess on her leg. The more purulent the abscess, the more the cancer regressed. It returned again when the abscess healed and regressed again when the abscess was reactivated.

Among the cures were soft-tissue sarcomas, neuroblastomas, melanomas and other types. Nauts noted that Native Americans have far lower death rates from cancer than people whose ancestors came later. But the Native American rate of parasite infestation and infection is 6 times greater. An alert immune system that is always fighting foreign invaders may serve us better.

Syphilis and malaria were said to regress cancer. Nauts wrote that in 1852 a physician advocated cancer prevention by infecting everyone with syphilis. He'd seen that prostitutes [presumably syphilitic] never had uterine cancer. With that in mind, he inoculated a woman who had inoperable breast cancer with pus from a syphilis chancre. The pain vanished while the cancer slowly disappeared. Then he cured the syphilis. But he advised not to use the treatment on terminal cancer patients.

The late cancer specialist Ewan Cameron wrote that a Dr. Coley, who practiced in the 1890s and early 1900s, also saw that a severe bacterial infection will regress certain cancers.[6] The body mobilizes its immune response to overcome the infection and the cancer, although not the primary target, is attacked as well by tumor necrosis factor [cachectin], a substance released from certain white cells.[7] This is an example of collateral damage as applied to healing rather than to civilian casualties in wartime. [Not all infections mobilise cachectin. Infection by *T. gondii* inhibits tumor growth in mice by drastically retarding the formation of new blood vessels that are needed for expansion.[8]]

In the late 1890s Coley began to inject bacterial toxins that caused the same effect as a severe bacterial infection.   [An organism he worked with, now known as *Serratia marcescens,* is generating renewed interest.]   Some Coley-method cure rates exceed those of today but its use declined and is now all but forgotten, having lost out to radiation early in the 20th century. A follow-up report on a group of patients 5 to 80 years after treatment with the method was presented at a London conference in 1978. The survival rate is impressive: 426 of 894 patients, of whom 237 had inoperable cancer.

Coley was made an Honorary Fellow of the Royal College of Surgeons in 1935, convincing evidence that physicians recognized the effectiveness of his method.   Yet less than 20 years later the American Cancer Society placed his method on what Cameron called a quackery list.[6] This was done because there has been no proof by scientific trial that Coley's injections are better than placebo shots.

Whenever a promising cancer treatment isn't lucrative enough to warrant funding for a scientific study it is buried along with all other cheap alternatives. We can understand why so many individuals sick with cancer are willing to try quack therapy. They're bothered by a suspicion that the establishment attempts to funnel all cancer victims into its own expensive programs, to the exclusion of present-day Dr. Coleys.

Quacks are adept at reinforcing that mistrust.   It has been rumored that some of them lace their secret concoctions with C, knowing it provides a lift to patients whose levels of it are bound to be low, first because of cancer and second because conventional therapy does not replenish the loss due to the stress of worry, radiation and toxic chemicals. Word gets around that the cancer patient down the street went to Dr. Elmallard and is now feeling much better. Soon growing numbers of desperate people are making the man rich.

Part of the blame falls on the specialists who fail to maintain the highest possible blood level of C after they've finished with chemotherapy and radiation. Doses greater than a gram a day were said to destroy free radicals that toxic treatments generate to kill cancer cells, therefore it is necessary to limit C intake during those treatments, according to an article in the lay press.[9]

This is as close as the establishment has come to admitting that C is antitoxic. Perhaps the complaint was also an attempt to eliminate competition. We should be extremely wary of negative statements about C. Its ability to cut viral nucleic acid might make it as effective against some cancers as toxic drugs, yet it would act only on the cancer without stressing the entire body.

A general statement about treatment for cancer is meaningless because of its many different types. The diversity calls for varied treatments. Extra C may be of value for some leukemias but not for others, for example. In leukemia-cell cultures of different types, C suppressed growth in 17% but accelerated it in 33%.[10] This is both good news and bad news if we assume the results would apply in actual therapy. One in six would benefit but twice as many would experience an opposite effect.

If a proprietary, patentable substance were shown to benefit 17% of cancer patients, researchers would receive funds from the government or a drug company to learn how to choose that group for treatment. A book was written about a proprietary drug that appeared to cure only 4% of certain cancer patients and retard growth in 12%.[11] High-dose C may do as well but, not being patentable, its usefulness will never be proved.

Herbs are not given much chance either, although some may be of value. Echinacea is worthy of notice. Varro Tyler, professor of pharmacology at Purdue University, wrote in *Herbs of Choice* [1994; Pharmaceutical Products Press, Binghampton, NY] that the herb causes the release of tumor necrosis factor. You'll recall it's the same substance certain white cells release to battle infection [page 40]. Tyler cautions that echinacea should not be used by anyone who has a severe systemic disease such as tuberculosis, collagen diseases, multiple sclerosis "and the like." By that he probably means autoimmune diseases such as lupus erythematosus.

Overall, cancer mortality has declined recently. Prostate- and breast-cancer therapy have improved.   But the prognosis is poor for oldsters with leukemia, lung or lymph cancer. A physician damped any optimistic outlook by noting that, except for a small group of cancer types, specialists practice mostly palliation. Whether the side effects of toxic chemotherapy can be called palliation is arguable. Even so, most of us would grasp the straw. When the future appears bleak we need to hope. If hope [treatment] is not offered, a specialist wrote, patients will get it from quacks.[12]

Now there's a revelation. It appears that predation on cancer patients is not limited to quacks. Specialists compete with them for the sale of hope. The only difference between the two may be in the degree of misery and who pays the bill. Quacks can't milk insurance or the government. The patient must pay---up front. Quack drugs are gentler, however. A doctor wrote that a specialist boasted of curing an aggressive cancer---but the patient soon died of damage due to toxic chemotherapy. The lessons learned from those toxic programs, I suppose, are not for us but for the benefit of our grandchildren.

The idea that C might retard the progress of some cancers, or even regress them, stems from early reports in the German literature and the observations of U.S. physicians. Edward Greer of Illinois wrote in 1954 about controlling myelogenous leukemia with up to 42 grams of C a day.[13] After Pauling's 1970 book about the common cold and one in 1976 that added flu to diseases that C could treat, in 1979 he and Ewan Cameron, a Scottish cancer specialist, published *Cancer and Vitamin C*.[14] An expanded edition appeared in 1993.[15]   They had written several scientific papers on cancer. The clinical work was done by Cameron.

Cameron had written a book in 1966 about how certain cancers overcome body resistance and expand. Resistance includes an active immune response and good strength in the tissue that surrounds a cancerous growth. This tissue, the intercellular cement, is laced with collagen. Collagen has been called the glue that holds us together. Several years ago a lecturer at a seminar said that if every substance except collagen were removed from our bodies, our friends would still recognize us.

Cameron thought of collagen as tissue reinforcement, like the metal rods in concrete. He noted that some malignant tumors produce enzymes, hyaluronidase and collagenase, that weaken the tissue around them, thereby allowing the cancer to expand easily. He expressed the hope that a way could be found to block those enzymes, strengthen the tissue around a cancer and boost the immune system.

A diet rich in C strengthens collagen substantially, as shown by experiments on guinea pigs, and supports a healthy immune system. Pauling, knowing that extra C causes increased production of a substance that inhibits the action of hyaluronidase, suggested that Cameron try it on cancer patients. Cameron was skeptical. He'd been treating the disease for years and had seen many plausible ideas come and go. But the patients who were classified as "untreatable" had nothing to lose, so in November, 1971, he began to give them extra C, usually 10 grams a day.

An ongoing disease can drain body reserves of C down to the prescurvy level. One should expect improvement when they are replenished, therefore the first benefits were seen in 5 to 10 days. Patients were more alert, had better appetites and less need for painkillers. Some were able to discontinue narcotics altogether, without experiencing withdrawal symptoms. The jaundiced condition improved in some; others could breathe easier; and a decreased red-cell sedimentation rate occurred, an indication of better response to the disease.

All of the above translates into a better quality of life. Dr. H.L. Newbold confirmed this in his book *Vitamin C Against Cancer* [1979; Stein & Day, New York]. He felt that cancer patients should consult a nutritionist as well as a specialist. A woman who had been reduced to exhaustion by chemotherapy and radiation came to his office for help. He returned her to an enjoyable state of living after 6 days of intravenous C and large oral doses thereafter. The regimen delayed advance of the cancer for several months.

"What would you do if you had cancer?" Newbold asked a scientist who had done survival-time comparisons and other statistical work at Memorial Sloan-Kettering and Roswell Park Memorial Institute for Cancer Research. The man replied that if it had metastasized he would try to live out his life as peacefully as possible. Newbold asked, "Without chemotherapy?" The man replied, "Without anything." It's an interesting comment from a person who had worked with survival figures for years. Let us hope that newer, benign drugs will elicit a more optimistic comment from today's statisticians.

Newbold questioned other physicians who'd been giving extra C to cancer patients. One who wished to remain anonymous said it was "absolutely super as a pain killer." His intravenous doses were 30 to 60 grams in a half liter of solution, dripped in over a period of 30 to 45 minutes. Archie Kalokerinos, an Australian physician, used that amount also, given 3 times a week, plus oral doses of 32 grams daily. Cancers were put on hold but not cured. It's about all conventional chemotherapy can do to most of them.

Now we've acquired background knowledge and broadened our perspective. The stage is set for another skirmish between C and its critics. Pauling again moved far out on a limb by stating that cancer incidence and mortality could be reduced by 75% with proper use of the vitamin. The co-founder of the Institute, Dr. Arthur B. Robinson, objected to such claims. Their relationship turned bitter over a disputed trial with mice. Robinson contended that the mice on C were developing more cancers than the controls. He said the dose of C must be almost lethal in order to arrest the growth of the cancers.

It could be argued that a near-lethal dose is a near-perfect definition of conventional chemotherapy. And that mice are not humans.

Pauling said he arrived at the 75% estimate by extrapolation from epidemiological data. In his defense, we must admit that no one has proved him wrong. There has been no trial in which thousands of participants used C properly all their lives while a control group's intake was limited to that obtained from their diet. In a good percentage of people this amount is less than the RDA.

Those are the ones who may run the greatest risk of developing cancer. A study reported in 2001 found that the lower the blood level of C in men, the greater the risk of death from all causes, including cancer. This held true for women also except for cancer.[16] Women usually have higher blood levels of C than men. It seems to tell us that a low C level is indeed a factor in the incidence of cancer.

In the Cameron/Pauling book on cancer, Cameron mentioned that at first he was skeptical about giving extra C to cancer patients. Later he became convinced that in some cases it is better than radiation or chemotherapy. He cited the following case in which C was given only as a substitute for doing nothing while the patient awaited his turn for conventional treatment:

A man, 42, was diagnosed as having reticulum cell sarcoma [now called histiocytic lymphoma]. Cameron stated that such cancers are deadlier than the Hodgkin's type, but treatable. The patient was to be transferred to Glasgow for radiation and chemotherapy when the facility had room for him. Meanwhile, he was to stay at the local hospital under Cameron's care. While he waited he was given 10 grams of C a day intravenously as palliation. Cameron stressed that the use of C had not been the treatment of choice. It was "...merely planned as a holding operation for this gravely ill man until conventional treatment would be available."

"The response was unexpectedly dramatic," Cameron continued. "Within less than two weeks all clinical manifestations of his disease had resolved, and his chest x-ray photographs rapidly returned to normal." On day 11 the C regimen was switched from intravenous to oral dosing, 10 grams of sodium ascorbate daily. On day 14 a trend toward cure was seen on the chest x-ray. Complete resolution occurred on day 22. The man was discharged with instructions to continue taking the oral dose until further notice. Two months later Cameron decided to taper it down to zero at the rate of 2.5 grams per month. Notice that the entire 10-gram regimen was not discontinued abruptly.

Four weeks after the dose reached zero, signs and symptoms of the lymphoma returned. The 10-gram daily oral regimen was resumed. It was not effective. The disease actually worsened during the next 2 weeks. The man was hospitalized and given 20 grams of C per day intravenously. Even at twice the dose of his first treatment the response was not immediate. For a few days Cameron wondered whether it would come at all. When it did come, the regression was rapid, so that at the end of 2 weeks the dose was switched to 12.5 grams orally. Upon discharge the man was told to continue the regimen indefinitely. X-ray evidence of the disease did not resolve completely for 5 months. Cameron reported details of the case in a professional journal in 1975.[17]

After more than 13 years on the regimen the man decided to discontinue it, against strong urgings not to. He said he wanted to know if he was really cured. He was still well 3 years later when Cameron submitted a report of the case for publication in the cancer journal *Oncology* [1991; 48:495-7]. Although experts on both sides of the Atlantic agreed that slides related to the case suggested a highly malignant lymphoma, the journal editor had 2 experts in London examine them before publication of the report. This was done, with no change in the diagnosis.

One would think that a successful treatment of lymphoma with C, reported first in 1975 and again in 1991, would prompt specialists all over the world to initiate trials or at least try the vitamin on their own lymphoma cases. Some may have done so but no account appears in the literature. We're led to suspect that key individuals in the system are willing to sacrifice patients rather than investigate C as an alternative to toxic drugs.

High-dose C is not a cancer cure-all, however. Advocates have never made such a claim. After Cameron had used it for a time he wrote of its limitations. Of 100 terminal cancer patients treated with it, 45 will benefit only a little or not at all. The growth may even accelerate in one. But 55 of those 100 will definitely benefit, to the extent listed below:

25 will see slower cancer growth---much slower in a few.
20 will see the growth halted---for years in a few.
10 will see the growth recede---one may appear to be cured.

During a 5-year period at the hospital where Cameron practiced, 126 lung-cancer patients were admitted for evaluation and treatment. Only 1 was judged to have a fair prognosis. The cancer was removed surgically. He was still living 5 years later. Of the remaining 125 patients, the ones assigned to radiation or chemotherapy were considered to have a "slightly better prognosis than the others." The others were given either narcotics or extra C. The average survival times provided by the 4 treatments are shown below:

70 who received only narcotics averaged...........68 days.
17 who received chemotherapy averaged...........90 days.
14 who received radiation averaged...................184 days.
24 who received high-dose C averaged..............187 days.

Only 1 of the 125 was still living 3.5 years later, still taking high-dose C.

In the book mentioned on page 42, usual chemotherapy was said to put breast cancers on hold for an average of about 4.6 months. Adding the new "breakthrough" drug extended the time by 3 months, on average. Extra C can do as well. There's no excuse for excluding it from cancer therapy. The reluctance to use it suggests a link to the earlier cold-trial mentality that excluded it from acceptance as a therapeutic substance in order to preserve the market for patentable drugs.

Cameron started his cancer patients on sodium ascorbate, given intravenously for 10 days before switching to an oral regimen, usually with the same dose. The good response in most patients convinced him that a clinical trial should be conducted but he felt he couldn't ethically withhold C from patients who would serve as a control group. Other cancer specialists at the hospital were not treating with C, however, so that a control group could be made up of their patients.

Pauling presented some early comparisons between the two groups to the National Cancer Institute and requested funds for a clinical trial. The request was denied. The American Cancer Society also turned him down. Not one to take no for an answer, he kept urging the National Cancer Institute to do something.

Meanwhile, the number of Cameron's C-treated patients approached 500, enough so that the records of 100 could be compared with the records of 1,000 patients who had not been given extra C. To eliminate selection bias, persons who had no interest in the outcome were assigned the job of matching one of Cameron's patients with 10 non-C patients treated by other specialists. The starting point for comparison was the day that the patient was judged untreatable, that further medication, or C, was given only as a palliative.

When the comparison was complete it was seen that patients who were given C lived about 4 times longer than their matched controls---an average of 210 days versus 50. An impressive 16% of C patients lived longer than a year, 50 times the percentage for the non-C group. This study was reported in 1976.[18]

Because of questions about whether both groups had been judged untreatable at comparable times in the course of the disease, a second study was done, with special attention paid to equalizing the starting point of the untreatable state. The difference, reported in 1978, was not significant but favored C slightly.[19] The C group's mean survival time was put at 300 days longer than those in the non-C group. In this later study, 22 of the 100 C patients [22%] were seen to have lived longer than a year, versus only 0.4% of non-C patients. The mean survival time of the 22 was 2.4 years. Eight were still alive at the time of the report, with a mean survival time of 3.5 years.

The above investigations were *retrospective* studies---a look back at the records of patients, most of whom had died before the study began. Such investigations are subject to bias. Although Cameron had not been involved in matching C with non-C patients, a retrospective study is not considered as reliable as a *prospective* study, in which the outcome at a future time is not considered to be subject to bias or manipulation. But keep in mind the statement quoted in the first chapter---about fraud in medical research being pervasive. Consider motives, such as who stands to gain financially.

For several years no government funds were available for a prospective clinical cancer trail to evaluate C but the spreading good news by Pauling and Cameron appeared to lubricate the grant machinery. The National Institutes of Health funded a trial by specialists at the Mayo Clinic. The results were reported in the *New England Journal of Medicine*, September 27, 1979, under this title:

FAILURE OF HIGH-DOSE VITAMIN C (ASCORBIC ACID) THERAPY TO BENEFIT PATIENTS WITH ADVANCED CANCER.

As with the hepatitis trial, [page 11], the outcome of this cancer trial was also revealed in the title. Busy doctors had no reason to read another word. Those who did read further could list several reasons for criticizing the study.   First, a selection bias was evident in that the study excluded leukemia cases, a convenient omission if the object was to discredit C. A leukemia patient in Cameron's C group lived almost 2.5 years after having been judged hopeless. Her matched control patients lived an average of 30 days. [The information gathered from a mouse study [p42] that C may either retard or accelerate the leukemic process was not known at the time of the study, therefore would not have been an excuse for excluding leukemia cases.]

Second, the Mayo patients were not started on intravenous doses as were Cameron's. Getting a quick start with IV C might have increased survival time significantly.   Third, only 4 of Cameron's 100 C patients had received chemotherapy during the treatable stage of their disease; and only 20 had received radiation. Nearly all of the 123 Mayo patients had been so treated, leaving only 4 or 5 patients in each arm of the trial [C and placebo group] who had not had radiation or chemotherapy. Those two traumas can interfere with the body's immune response.

Fourth, some of the 63 non-C patients could have been taking C surreptitiously. Urinary C was checked, just once, in only 5 from that group, chosen at random, according to a letter to the journal by 2 members of the research team [Jan. 31, 1980]. At least one patient in the non-C group is a prime suspect. He had not responded to "many previous attempts at chemotherapy." But he lived longer than all the others. A record of that sort tells us that we should never underestimate the power of a placebo.

Or perhaps high-dose C.

Meanwhile, Japanese scientists were also studying the effects of C on terminal cancer patients. Their principal report, an update of an earlier one in 1978, was published in 1982.[20] Low doses, not more than a gram a day, were tried initially. Dosing with larger amounts began in 1974. By 1977 daily doses of 30 grams or more were being given, some intravenously, and compared with doses of 4 grams a day or less.

The high-dose group lived 5.6 times longer, on average, than the low-dose group. Patients who took 4 grams or less per day lived 43 days after being judged hopeless. Similar patients, whose daily intake ranged from 5 to more than 30 grams a day, lived 246 days. Three were "clinically well" and still living at the time of the report, averaging 1,550 days of life. Their cancers, of breast, thymus and uterus, were still in place but not active.

The investigators noted that in this study C was "especially effective for cancer of the uterus, whereas it gives smaller increase in survival time for cancer of the stomach and lung than for other kinds of cancer." [As you may know, cancer of the uterine cervix is associated with a virus.] They found that doses higher than 30 grams a day were less effective. The reason, they thought, was that those patients were sicker.

Extra C was of benefit to hopeless patients at another hospial also. Those on 5 to 30 grams a day averaged 67 days more life than those on placebo. Although the number of patients was small, interesting information emerged. A patient with bladder cancer on high-dose C was still living at the time of the report, 215 days and counting. In 3 months the tumor had decreased in volume from 115 to 7 [the unit of measurement was not given]. And while only 1 of 6 patients on high-dose C needed narcotics to control pain, 15 of the 19 on placebo needed the drugs.

Because of criticism of their first trial, Mayo cancer specialists received another government grant for a second one. None of the patients had had prior chemotherapy but they still differed from Cameron's group in that only cancers originating in the colon or rectum were involved, a disease with no known treatment at the time. Cameron's study included cancers of 16 different organs.

Again the results of the Mayo study were reported in the *New England Journal of Medicine*, January 17, 1985. High-dose C was shown to be of no value in the treatment of advanced cancer, indicating that whether patients had had prior chemotherapy was not a factor in the outcome.

The report was accompanied by an editorial from an official in the National Cancer Institute who wrote: "It is difficult to find fault with the design or execution of this study." He endeavored to discourage any further investigation of C by adding "...trials with other types of tumor do not appear warranted."

Three heavy guns had blasted C back into limbo: Mayo Specialists, Big Man in the National Cancer Institute and Prestigious Medical Journal. We suspect they were mighty proud of the way they had shot C down, and with words so piously delivered that we might also suspect they were genuinely saddened to contemplate results not in favor of C.

Let us read more than just the title and abstract of the report. Colorectal-cancer patients were chosen because, there being no known treatment, it would not be unethical to have an untreated control group. And it was pointed out that Cameron's patients with the disease had done well on high-dose C. The Mayo patients, unlike Cameron's, were not started on intravenous C, however.

We flip a couple pages to look at Figure 1, lines representing survival times of C and placebo groups.....rather interesting.....at no time did the C-group line show that they were outliving the placebo group. Percentagewise, they had died *sooner* than those who had not been taking C.

Why had that happened? In previous reports, groups that took C outlived non-C groups. In the first Mayo trial, for example, the "survival lines" show that at any point in time, except for 3 instances in the final weeks, more C patients were living than placebo patients [those 3 may have been taking C surreptitiously]. Why had this second trial shown an opposite effect?

A reading of the abstract offered no clue. A careful reading of the rest of the report might turn up something.....Ah-yes.....In the small-print section that details trial procedure we come upon it. One sentence stands out to reveal how the beneficial effect of extra C had been crippled. It states: "Therapy was continued as long as the patient was able to take oral medication or until there was evidence of marked progression of the malignant disease."

In other words, the C intake was discontinued abruptly in mid-trial---*even though the patient was able to take it!*

Compare the above quote with one in the first trial report: "Treatment was continued until death or until the patient was no longer able to take oral medication." In that respect the first Mayo trial followed Cameron's procedure. The second trial did not.

Cameron had written in the journal *Cancer Research* [1979; 39:663-81] that high doses of C should be continued as long as possible, that stopping it might cause a "brisk reactivation" of the cancer. He had passed along this important observation, then saw it callously employed to discredit his research!

The definition of *terminal* as it applies to cancer patients [of or in the final stages of a fatal disease] implies a period of decline. The purpose of the trial was to determine whether large doses of C could retard the decline. Stopping the dose while patients could still take it converted the trial into a subtle vehicle for discrediting C.

For that purpose it was quite effective. When you read in so many publications that C has been scientifically shown to be of no value in cancer therapy you can be sure the writers were thoroughly bamboozled by experts who knew that very few readers possessed enough background knowledge to suspect trickery.

The trial was a piece of junk. Perhaps its only value is the demonstration that abruptly discontinuing a high dose of C is detrimental. Patients abruptly deprived of C lived a mean of 2.9 months afterward. Those abruptly deprived of placebo lived a mean of 4.1 months, more than 40% longer.

Did the Mayo specialists realize that a high dose of C should not be stopped abruptly? Did they know of Cameron's paper that contained the warning? They couldn't help but know! They had listed the paper as a reference in their first trial report! And there are other comments in the literature about the hazard of abruptly discontinuing a high dose. In general, abrupt stoppage of medication is not common practice.

This is a good time to recall the words of skeptics who said we will learn the truth about C from results of scientific trials. Have we found any truth? The word *phony* is said to have derived from an old term for gilded brass rings claimed by con artists to be solid gold. Brass is doubly appropriate here, as in not genuine and as in a brazen lack of shame.

The comforting trust we should have for cancer-treatment institutions is weakened substantially by the realization that information gathered in some of them may be distorted by bias.

There are additional eyebrow-raisers connected with the second Mayo trial. This statement is found in the report: "...in our opinion there is no known form of chemotherapy for colorectal cancer that has been demonstrated to produce substantive palliative benefit or extension of survival." Now note this statement on the folowing page: "Somewhat more than half the patients who have discontinued participation in this study (58 of 98) have received subsequent chemotherapy." The number of former C and placebo patients who shared that useless trauma and waste of healthcare funds was about equal. This is the employment of treatment in response to a patient's hope, a commodity that specialists sell in competition with quacks.

After publication of the first trial report in the *New England Journal of Medicine* in 1979, later issues of the journal printed 8 letters of criticism or comment about the trial. Letters by both Pauling and Cameron appeared. After publication of the second trial report the journal did not publish a single letter relating to the trial. Surely criticism of the "members of the club" who trashed C would have been as sharp as that generated by the first trial report. But the editor, the gatekeeper member of the trashing group, had slammed the gate against those who wrote to point out how the trial had deviated from Cameron's procedure.

Incidentally, the trial-report issue of the journal contained 56 pages of medical articles and 97 pages of advertising, mostly pharmaceutical.

In his book *How to Live Longer and Feel Better,* the 1987 softcover edition by Avon, Pauling referred to the trial as a fraud [p 313]. He also noted that none of the patients on C died while taking the high dose [p 234]. In the Pauling Institute *Newsletter* of spring/summer 1985, he faulted the researchers for using a lactic-acid placebo. A participant can open a capsule, taste it, determine it is not C, then switch to the treatment group. Pauling wrote: "It is difficult to understand why experienced clinical researchers would spend public funds for a second study without assuring themselves that the protocol they planned to use was appropriate for obtaining the stated objective."

Some of the researchers involved in the study with C and colorectal cancer were also investigating another substance, levamisole, as treatment for the disease. One may wonder if they would have preferred to see high-dose C, advocated by Pauling and Cameron, or their drug levamisole to be be the treatment of choice for the cancer. As it turned out, levamisole was promoted by the system for a time but was seen to be no better than any other drug.[21]

Levamisole, used mainly as a livestock dewormer when first marketed, sold for a few cents a pill. Its price was 100 times greater when sold as a cancer drug. To the Mayo group's credit, one of them blasted the drug company for the gouge. When you watch those honey-oozing "we care" ads by pharmaceutical companies bear in mind that they're in business for the money, not for sympathetic reasons. In general they do an excellent job and are well compensated, as they should be. But no one at the top really cares enough to allow high-dose C its proper place in cancer therapy. And if the FDA didn't resist their pressure and exercise a modicum of control occasionally, prescription drugs as the fourth leading cause of death probably would move up to third or second.

Consumers Union, publisher of the informative and usually objective *Consumer Reports*, published several editions of the book *The New Medicine Show.* Chapter 14 of the 6th edition, 1989, contains 2 paragraphs about C and cancer. Identical comments may have appeared in other editions. It is stated in the first paragraph that Cameron's study was not properly designed. In what way was not mentioned. Paragraph 2 contains 3 sentences, the last of which compares C and placebo groups in the Mayo studies. "The researchers found no differences in survival time, appetite, severity of pain, weight loss, or amount of nausea and vomiting." Note that difference in strength is not mentioned.

Patients in the second Mayo trial were not on C long enough to have differed from those on placebo. The above quote refers to the first trial report, which contains a table showing those differences, except for weight, which appears in the abstract. Listed in that table, along with the other comparisons, is *strength*. Of the patients in the C group, 26% exhibited greater strength, versus 13% in the placebo group. In other words, twice as many C patients were stronger, a 100% difference in favor of C. The C patients were favored by 60% less pain also.

To omit mention of the difference in strength and state that no difference was seen in the amount of pain indicates bias against C on the part of the medical advisers to Consumers Union. Both the editors and the public were misled. A reduction in pain while taking high-dose C is nearly always noted by physicians who use it in cancer management. You'll recall the Japanese study [page 52] in which 15 of 19 patients [79%] on placebo needed narcotics versus only 1 of 6 [17%] in the C group.

Besides boosting nutrition, collagen and immune strength while easing pain and inhibiting tumor enzymes that weaken surrounding tissue, does extra C do any more to combat cancer? Does it attack the cancer directly? The following 2 case histories detailed in the Cameron/Pauling book *Cancer and Vitamin C* lead us to suspect that it does. C can either attack some cancers directly or mount a phenomenal immune response. Note:

The testicular cancer of a man continued to spread throughout his body even after removal of a testicle and radiation treatment. When seen at a later date metastatic colonies of cancer cells were thriving in many areas, including a large mass on the gum of the upper jaw. His condition was hopeless.

He was hospitalized and started on 8 grams of C per day intravenously. Less than 2 days later the large mass on the upper gum had broken down and was bleeding profusely. The C infusion was stopped but the man's condition began to deteriorate. He died about 2 weeks later.

Extensive metastatic areas were seen in the lungs, brain and abdomen at autopsy. Cameron wrote: "...the striking feature was that all these metastases were dead, and could be easily scooped out." Extra C had killed the cancer colonies so quickly that the blood vessels supplying them had no time to shut down. In the brain such a condition translates into a massive stroke.

A few months later a man who had lived for 5 years aided by chemotherapy and hormone treatments after removal of a cancerous kidney had deteriorated to a hopeless condition when hospitalized. Cancer colonies were well established in many organs. He was started on 10 grams of C per day orally. Within 36 hours this man also exhibited signs of a stroke. He lapsed into a coma and died 3 days later. In Cameron's oral regimen the 10 grams were divided into 4 doses of 2.5 grams each, suggesting that the man had taken only 15 grams of C before deteriorating.

The 2 cases were among the first that Cameron treated with C, at a time when he was still low on the learning curve. The unfortunate outcomes taught him to begin the first day of C therapy with only a gram, then increase by a gram a day until the treatment amount was reached. This gradual approach prevented any further bleeding complications.

One of the most ridiculous attempts to belittle C appeared in a family medical book several years ago. An overdone list of side effects included a warning that it shrinks cancers too rapidly. No mention of any good from extra C appeared.

Several cancer case histories showing benefit from C follow. Most appear in the Pauling/Cameron book on the subject.

A physician's wife began to notice she was writing erratically. During the following 2 months her right arm, leg and facial muscles weakened somewhat and she had difficulty speaking and swallowing. A brain scan revealed a tumor about an inch in diameter. Her husband and 2 neurosurgeons advised immediate surgery, which would leave her with a partially paralyzed arm and leg.

The frightening prospect drove her to try 10 grams of C a day, a regimen that a relative recalled reading something about. A few weeks later she noticed a return of strength to the affected muscles. A brain scan indicated that the tumor was breaking up. Two months later a scan showed no evidence of the tumor. Its only residual effect was said to be a slight droop in the corner of her mouth.

"Spontaneous regression," a neurosurgeon announced.

Such is the lot of vitamin C---to be brushed off without a nod of recognition.

The mesothelium, a cover tissue of lungs, intestines and heart, can fall prey to a cancer called mesothelioma. It's a favorite for asbestos-related lung cancer. Upon being diagnosed with this type of cancer, a woman put it on hold by taking 10 grams of C a day. She was leading an archeological expedition at the time of Cameron's report.

A man, 40, was treated with steroids and blood transfusions over a period of 2 years for a condition misdiagnosed as aplastic anemia. When a bone-marrow biopsy indicated chronic lympho-cytic leukemia the steroids were discontinued. They had caused osteoporosis, with resultant small fractures of the vertebrae. Transfusions were still necessary---6 to 8 pints every 5 or 6 weeks. He decided to skip radiation and chemotherapy and treat himself with high-dose C---35 grams a day. He began to feel better. At the time of the report he no longer needed transfusions and was building a new house for his new life.

A 67-year-old man had part of his stomach and nearby lymph nodes removed to eliminate most of the cancer in the area. His daughter, a nurse, put him on 12 grams of C a day. Within 6 months the cancer returned. He was hospitalized and, deprived of C, began to fail rapidly. Removing him from the hospital, his daughter started him on 20 grams of C a day, then gradually built up to 28 grams. His dramatic return to better health suggests that the dose should be as high as possible. At surgery for gallstones 16 months later, no sign of cancer was seen.

During an 18-month period a woman, 47, had surgery for bilateral ovarian cancer; a second surgery to clear intestinal adhesions; a third to clear a cancerous bowel obstruction; and a fourth to establish a colostomy. Given 6 months to live, she was started on chlorambucil, a mild chemotherapy drug. On her own she began to take C, up to 12 grams a day, as much as the bowel would tolerate. Chlorambucil was discontinued 20 months later but she kept taking extra C. She was alive and well 6 years later.

A woman of 49 was started on radiation after removal of a cancerous breast. Armpit lymph nodes were removed 2 years later and hormone therapy begun. A year passed before neck nodes were removed; and 13 months later cancerous ovaries had to go. She was put on 10 grams of C a day. Still living 7 years after the first surgery.

A man bleeding from nose and rectum was almost bedridden when he learned he had multiple myeloma. Before starting chemotherapy he took extra C, quickly raising to 40 grams a day, all the bowel would tolerate. In 5 days the rectal bleeding stopped. As recovery progressed the bowel began to signal with diarrhea that he no longer needed so much C. Dose reduction in line with body needs continued until stabilizing at 20 grams a day. Blood analysis 10 months later was normal and biopsy of the bone marrow showed no evidence of the disease.

Recently, nucleic acid from a herpes virus has been detected in the bone marrow of myeloma patients. Oddly, the viral material was found in the healthy dendritic cells, not in cancerous plasma cells. The virus is said to make the healthy cells produce a substance that promotes malignancy.[22]

The book contains many more encouraging examples of the value of extra C in the management of cancer.

An 81-year-old man's account of his experience with colon cancer appears in the *Linus Pauling Institute Newsletter*, winter of 1985-6. He'd had surgery for the condition 5 years before. At the time it had metastasized to the liver but a heart condition ruled out more surgery. He was started on chemotherapy but a reading of the medical literature on the subject convinced him that treatment of colon cancer was useless. The cancerous mass in the liver actually increased by 50% while he was on the drug.

He wrote to the Pauling Institute for information. Pauling suggested he begin with 12 grams of C a day and increase to 25 gradually. Instead, the man moved the daily dose up to 36 grams, to the "edge of diarrhea," and added 50 mcg of selenium, some vitamin E and other vitamins and minerals to the regimen. His next scan revealed that the mass in the liver had not enlarged. X-ray findings 18 months after the first surgery showed that a lump below the breast bone had vanished. Later, ultrasound images indicated that the liver mass was shrinking.

For some reason he stopped taking magnesium and vitamin E but resumed when the cancer began to grow again. His latest scan, 5 years and 2 months after bowel surgery, suggested a stable cancer that was calcifying, a good sign, and clear lungs, also a good sign because bowel cancers metastasize to the liver first, then to the lungs. An additional benefit from the regimen was protection from colds and flu, even though he deliberately associated with friends when they had the diseases.

His greatest wonderment was that none of the dozen physicians he knew were interested in how he had managed to live so long with such a malignant disease.

Abram Hoffer, a Canadian psychiatrist who treated with a regimen that included high-dose C, wrote of 3 cancer cases in the spring, 1981 *Linus Pauling Institute Newsletter*: An old man with a mental problem had terminal bronchial cancer for which he had received radiation. He was put on high-dose C and 3 grams of niacin per day. The mental problem resolved in 3 days. No cancer was seen on x-ray film at a later date. He lived for 28 months before dying of heart disease.

The mother of a 15-year-old girl with malignant sarcoma in an arm was urged to consent to amputation. Instead, the girl was put on high-dose C and other vitamins. When Hoffer wrote of the case she had been well for more than 10 years.

A jaundiced woman with inoperable cancer of the pancreas started herself on 10 grams of C a day. Her doctor referred her to Hoffer, who raised the C intake to 40 grams, added other nutrients and advised a better diet. No tumor was seen at the time of her last check-up. Unfortunately, such therapy does not help everyone, Hoffer wrote. There are failures also.

Hoffer and Pauling started a book on cancer and vitamin C that Hoffer finished and published under his name after the death of Pauling. Title: *Vitamin C & Cancer* Discovery Recovery Controversy [2000; Quarry Press, Kingston, Ontario, Canada]. Although the edition lacks an index, the material is encouraging and the contents page is useful.

Physicians at the University of Basel in Switzerland have used high-dose C in cancer therapy. A man with inoperable cancer of the bronchus regained weight and returned to work after being put on 15 grams of C a day. A recurrent tumor of the head and neck regressed after 14 grams of C a day. And high-dose C plus interferon regressed a recurrent breast cancer.[23] [Extra C causes the body to increase production of its own interferon.]

A retired physician who in 1996 had colon cancer involving at least 1 lymph node wrote me in 1999. He rejected chemotherapy in favor of 30 or more grams of C dripped in intravenously 3 times a week at first then once a week for 18 months, then 12 to 18 grams a day orally. The cancer had not returned.

The anticancer activity of C is potentiated by attaching phosphorus to it, providing more of the antioxidant to cells resisting the spread of mouse melanoma.[24] And vitamin K_3 teams with C to kill cancer cells without harming normal ones.[25] Discoveries of this sort are changing the establishment mindset in areas where it counts. In 2000, Scientists at the National Institutes of Health wrote: "It is time to review ascorbate's efficacy as an anticancer agent, when administered intravenously in large doses, as reported in the studies by Cameron, Campbell and Pauling." [26]

If extra C can regress certain cancers it should be able to suppress them earlier---even prevent them. People who eat more C-rich food have less cancer. A review of the evidence by Gladys Block makes a strong case for eating such foods or taking extra C.[27] Amounts needn't be huge; only 500 mg 3 times a day will prevent harmful chemical reactions in the urinary bladder that lead to cancer.[28] And people who took 2 grams a day, along with zinc and other vitamins **halved** the recurrence rate of bladder cancer over those who took only the RDA.[29] How strange: we often read that extra C passes out in the urine without doing any good while word of this particular good is seldom printed!

If a cancer is initiated by a virus, larger amounts of C can prevent it by controlling the virus. Hepatitis C is said to be the "single most important risk factor" in the development of liver cancer. Hepatitis B is suspected also.[30, 31] Viruses are said to cause 15% of all cancers. The figure may rise as more is learned about causes. Uterine cervical cancer is associated with a virus. It is associated with smoking also[32] but probably secondarily because smoking lowers the blood level of C.

A relatively small intake of C appears to affect the occurrence of uterine cervical cancer. Women whose "pap" test revealed precancerous tissue change were seen to have only *half* the level of C found in women with normal tissue.[33] Another study separated women into 2 groups according to the amount of C in their diet. The intake was adequate in one group but provided less than half the RDA in the other. **Ten times** more women in the low-C group had precancerous tissue change.[34]

What do the study results appear to tell us? Would maintaining a higher blood level of C prevent most cervical cancers? Is the solution as simple as that? It seems logical because most of those cancers are associated with a virus. Experts who are searching for a high-tech solution can argue forever that the study results do not *prove* a connection. But they cannot contend the matter is not worth investigating.

Don't count on it ever being done, though. There's no financial advantage in proving a preventive role for C. Just the opposite, in fact. Testing, removing precancerous tissue and treating aggressively when the deteriorating body calls for help are all good money makers. By ignoring this good evidence the authorities appear to be thinking: *Go ahead, ladies, get that cancer! We're ready to help in your time of need---with surgery, radiation and whatever, to the outermost reach of our research horizons! .....Your insurance will cover it.*

Others will attend to last rites.

After completing the experiments that led to the conquest of yellow fever, Walter Reed wrote: "The prayer that...I might be permitted in some way or at some time to do something to alleviate human suffering has been granted!" The noble ethic is not always with us now. There seems to have been a complete abandonment of the moral obligation to explore without bias the tremendous potential of extra C.

References

1 Benade L, Howard T, Burk D. Synergistic killing of Ehrlich ascites carcinoma cells by ascorbic acid and 3-amino-1,2,4,-triazole. *Oncology* 1969; 23:33-43

2 Radetsky P. Got cancer killers? *Discover* 1999; 20 (6):68-75

3 McCarthy M. Targeted drugs take centre stage at U.S. cancer meeting. *Lancet* 2001; 357:1593.

4 Seppa N. Leukemia overpowers drug in two ways. *Science News* 2001; 159:389.

5 Christensen D. New drug takes on intestinal cancer. *Science News* 2001; 159:328.

6 *Cancer and Vitamin C* Cameron E, Pauling L. 1979; The Linus Pauling Institute of Science and Medicine, Menlo Park, CA

7 Carswell E A, Old L J, Kassel R L, et al. An endotoxin serum factor that causes necrosis of tumors. *Proc Natl Acad Sci USA* 1975; 72:3666-70

8 Senior K. Infection seems to block angiogenesis in tumors. *Lancet* 2001; 357:1507.

9 Article in *Time* April 10, 2000 p146

10 Park C H. Biological nature of the effect of ascorbic acid on the growth of human leukemic cells. *Cancer Research* 1985; 45:3969-73

11 Payer L. A promising drug for breast cancer (book review). *Lancet* 1999; 353:334

12 Moertel S G. Current concepts in cancer chemotherapy: chemotherapy of gastrointestinal cancer. *N Engl J Med* 1978; 299:1049-52

13 Greer E. Alcoholic cirrhosis complicated by polycythemia vera and then myelogenous leukemia and tolerance of large doses of vitamin C. *Med Times* 1954; 82:865-8

14 *Cancer and Vitamin C*. Cameron E, Pauling L. 1979 Linus Pauling Institute of Science and Medicine, Menlo Park, California.

15 *Cancer and Vitamin C* Cameron E, Pauling L. 1993 Camino Pub Co. Phila

16 Khaw K T, Bingham S, Welch A, et al. Relation between plasma ascorbic acid and mortality in men and women in EPIC-Norfolk prospective study: a prospective population study. *Lancet* 2001; 357:657-63

17 Cameron E, Campbell A, Jack T. The orthomolecular treatment of cancer. III. Reticulum cell sarcoma: double complete regression induced by high-dose ascorbic acid therapy. *Chem Biol Interact* 1975; 11:387-93

18 Cameron E, Pauling L. Supplemental ascorbate in the supportive treatment of cancer: prolongation of survival times in terminal human cancer. *Proc Natl Acad Sci USA* 1976; 73:3685-9

19 Cameron E, Pauling L. Supplemental ascorbate in the supportive treatment of cancer: reevaluation of prolongation of survival times in terminal human cancer. *Proc Natl Acad Sci USA* 1978; 75:4538-42

20 Murata A, Morishige F, Yamaguchi H. Prolongation of survival times of terminal cancer in patients by administration of large doses of ascorbate. *Internatl J Vit Nutr Res* 1982; 23 Supp: 103-13.

21 Midgley R, Kerr D. Colorectal cancer (seminar) *Lancet* 1999; 353:391-9

Chapter 3 references

22 Rettig M B, Ma H J, Vescio R A, et al. Kaposi's sarcoma--associated herpesvirus infection of bone marrow dendritic cells from multiple myeloma patients. *Science* 1997; 276:1851-4

23 Hanck A. Tolerance and effects of high-doses of ascorbic acid. *Internatl J Vit Nutr Res* 1982; 23 supp:221-39, in *Vitamin C New Clinical Applications in Immunology, Lipid Metabolism and Cancer* 1982 Hanck A. Ed. Hans Huber Publishers. Bern. Stuttgart, Vienna

24 Nagao N, Nakayama T, Etoh T, et al. Tumor invasion is inhibited by phosphorylated ascorbate via enrichment of intracellular vitamin C and decreasing of oxidative stress. *J Cancer Res Clin Oncol* 2000; 126:511-18

25 Raloff J. Coming to terms with death: Accurate descriptions of a cell's demise may offer clues to diseases and treatments. *Science News* 2001; 159:378-80

26 Padayatty S J, Levine M. Reevaluation of ascorbate in cancer treatment: emerging evidence, open minds and serendipity. *J Am Coll Nutr* 2000; 19:423-5

27 Block G. Vitamin C and cancer prevention: the epidemiologic evidence *Am J Clin Nutr* 1991; 53:270s-82s

28 Schlegel J U, Pipkin G E, Nishimura R, Duke G A. Studies in the etiology and prevention of bladder carcinoma. *J Urol* 1969; 101:317-24

29 Lamm D L, Riggs D R, Shriver J S, et al. Megadose vitamins in bladder cancer: a double-blind clinical trial. *J Urol* 1994; 151:21-6

30 De Mitri M S, Poussin K, Baccarini P, et al. HCV-associated liver cancer without cirrhosis. *Lancet* 1995; 345:413-5

31 Hayden G H, Jarvis L M, Simmonds P, Hayes P C. Association between chronic hepatitis C and hepatocellular carcinoma. *Lancet* 1995; 345:928-9

32 Szarewski A, Jarvis M J, Sasieni P. et al. Effect of smoking cessation on cervical lesion size. *Lancet* 1996; 347:941-3

33 Romney S L, Duttagupta C, Basu J, et al. Plasma vitamin C and uterine cervical dysplasia. *Am J Obs Gyn* 1985; 151:976-80

34 Wasserthiel-Smoller S, Romney S L, Wylie-Rosett J. et al. Dietary vitamin C and uterine cervical dysplasia. *Am J Epidemiol* 1981; 144:714

4

Inadequate Dosing In Other Studies

A cause for concern in people with a genetic tendency to develop large numbers of colon polyps is the possibility that some may turn cancerous. The multiple-polyp condition can be a single affliction or part of a combination along with skin growths and bone tumors called *Gardner's syndrome.* Treatment of the bowel problem involves nipping out or electrically burning down the polyps. Sometimes the affected length of gut is removed or bypassed to prevent development of cancer, which is probably due to constant irritation of the polyps by bowel contents.

Investigators in 1975 cited evidence that in areas where colon cancer is more common, intestines of the inhabitants contain greater numbers of certain bacteria which remove hydrogen ions from bile acids. This created substances that could cause cancer. It was thought that supplying more hydrogen ions to the gut might block this transfer from the bile, thereby reducing the number of cancers.

Vitamin C readily gives up some hydrogen ions. Whether this generous act was the reason for fewer new polyps in 4 of 5 patients when they took 3 grams of C a day is not known for sure but the results generated other studies with C versus colon polyps. We'll look at the important ones.

In this first study mentioned,[1] all 5 patients had been diagnosed with familial polyposis. Surgeries for the condition were far enough in the past to be eliminated as a factor in the outcome of the study. Each took a gram of timed-release C 3 times a day. Some patients reported that not all the C dissolved before being eliminated, therefore the effective dose was somewhat less than 3 grams.

Case 1: A woman with a long history of polyp formation and previous surgery had 30 polyps removed in 1973. In 1974 29 new ones were seen; and removed, presumably, though not mentioned, so that the number would be zero at the start of the C regimen. After 6 months on C, 2 polyps were seen; and 6 at month 7. But only 2 were seen at month 10; and none at month 13. A stool sample contained 5 times more C than a control sample.

Case 2: In 1973 a man who'd had surgery 17 years before and regular removal of polyps since, had 25 removed. In 1974 the count was 45. Removal was not mentioned. He began taking 3 grams of C a day. At month 2 the count was 43; at month 4 it was 21; and down to 17 at month 6.

Case 3: A woman with the usual history had 2 of 12 polyps removed in 1974 before starting the C regimen. At month 2 only 2 small polyps were seen. The count was zero at month 4.

Case 4: A woman who'd had surgery in 1954 and yearly polyp removal for 9 years afterward enjoyed a period of remission until 1971, when a single polyp was removed. Six were removed in late 1973; 12 the following April; and 9 in late 1974. One was removed, so that 8 remained at the start of the 3-gram C regimen. At month 2 the count was down to 5 and at month 4 only 2 remained.

Case 5: A man had surgery in 1968 to remove part of the colon, which contained more than 200 polyps. For a short time afterward several polyps were removed every 2 months, then none was seen for 18 months. In January 1974, 4 were removed; and 12 in March. In September the count was 15 when he began taking 3 grams of C a day. The dose was ineffective. Polyp count had increased to 28 at month 6.

The 80% response rate from a moderate intake of 3 grams a day is impressive. Polyp numbers follow a wax-and-wane pattern that can skew the results of short-term studies but the range while on C for 30 months was less than usual. Whether higher' doses of C would have produced even more impressive results is not known. Higher doses were not tried.

Researchers in 1977 reported examining 280 members of 11 families with an inherited susceptibility to Gardner's syndrome.[2] Nearly half, 126, had one or more of the three conditions that comprise the syndrome. Ten with polyps were given 3 grams of C a day during the study. A brief account of the results:

Two had no change in size or number of polyps while on C.
Two had fewer polyps but no change in size.
Two had fewer and smaller polyps.
One had no change in number but polyps were smaller.
One had 4 polyps at start and none at month 7.
One had 24 polyps at start and 23 at month 5.
One had many polyps at start, none at month 3. Shortly after C was discontinued, 3 polyps were seen in this individual.
Size and number increased in 2 others after stopping C.

Final score: 8 of 10 benefited from extra C. Perhaps it could be said that all did, because none exhibited an increase in polyp number and size while on the regimen.

In a randomized controlled trial reported in 1982, 19 polyp-prone patients took 3 grams of C a day while 17 took placebo. After 9 months a trend toward polyp reduction was seen and after 18 months the total polyp area, as compared with the placebo group, had been reduced substantially. The authors concluded, however, that C has "no current therapeutic value."[3]

Doubling or tripling the dose might have changed their minds.

Even though practicing physicians had reported using much higher amounts of C in various treatments, researchers usually expressed concern over side effects that were thought to occur at doses beyond 3 grams. It is not clear whether this was a real hazard in their minds or an artificial one in the form of a road-block to publication of a paper. Researchers couldn't help but know that journal editors reject papers that report dramatic benefits from extra C. Less dramatic results had a better chance of being accepted.

What *is* clear is that 3 studies, one a controlled trial, had used 3 grams of C a day to reduce the number of colon polyps. The good news would prompt other physicians to try it, perhaps at much higher doses that might result in greater reductions. A seasoned reader of the literature on C would expect that fear of this happening would lead to a scientific trial which would show no benefit in order to discourage further investigation.

True to the observer's expectation, negative results from such a study were reported in 1988. It was so very difficult to raise the daily dose beyond 3 grams---but behold how easily it can be cut! The patients on C were not given the 3 grams [3,000 mg] per day that had been shown to be effective. Their daily dose was only 400 mg, a 7.5-fold reduction! To further fuzzy up the evaluation, 400 mg of vitamin E were given also. This exercise in evasion resulted in only a slight benefit over controls.[4]

A 1989 report: a daily 4 grams of C, 400 mg of E and 2.2 grams of fiber [bran] was compared with the same vitamin dose but 10 times the fiber [22.5 grams]. Controls took 60 mg of C, 2.2 grams of fiber, 4,000 units of A and about 60% of the RDA for other vitamins and minerals. The high-fiber, high-C group had fewer polyps but more diarrhea than the other two groups. The control group fared poorly for 30 months, then their polyp picture improved to equal the low-fiber, high C group.[5] [Perhaps the controls achieved equality by switching to C after tasting their placebo---it contained lactose rather than citric acid.]

A daily gram of C, 70 mg of vitamin E and 70,000 IU of vitamin A, reported in 1992, showed some benefit.[6] Another that used the same regimen was reported in 1993. Of those who took vitamins, 5.7% developed new polyps. Of those who took placebo, 35.9% developed new polyps.[7]

The trend toward encouraging results with C plus other vitamins led to a large-scale study involving 6 medical centers in the U. S. [The larger the number of patients, the greater the impression that research is of higher quality, regardless of the size of the dose.] The *New England Journal of Medicine* reported the results in 1994 [331:141-7] and fed the news to the Associated Press. Headlines blared that vitamins A, C and E cannot prevent cancers, as shown by their failure to prevent colon polyps. A physician was quoted as saying that lots of money is being spent to promote the idea that extra vitamins are cancer stoppers.

C advocates would contend that more money is being spent by his camp on trials with inadequate doses. How many readers would know that the meager gram a day used was far too low?

The vitamin E dose was 400 mg and beta carotene 25 mg, no more than normal. And none of the patients had the large numbers of polyps seen in familial polyposis. These were just people who'd had at least 1 polyp removed within 3 months of the start of the study. [Attitudes toward vitamins have improved recently. Although ineffective against lung cancer, vitamin E and selenium cut prostate cancer 20% during a study, prompting a new 12-year trial by the National Cancer Institute.]

The white cells of healthy folk have 38% more C than those in polyp formers, a percentage that applies to patients with other chronic diseases also.[8] Advocates who know C well are not surprised by the finding. Low C levels in sick people are usual. And are usually disregarded, thereby hindering recovery.

Idiopathic thrombocytopenic purpura [ITP] is an autoimmune disease in which the body's immune system attacks blood platelets [thrombocytes], reducing their numbers so that there aren't enough to prevent bleeding areas in the skin and elsewhere. A report that purpura regressed when *H. pylori* bacteria were cleared from the stomach[9] suggests that either the bacteria lower blood C level or that platelets and *H. pylori* have something in common that causes the immune system to attack both.

Usual treatments for ITP include corticosteroids; anticancer drugs; immune suppressants; intravenous gammaglobulin; and spleen removal. A 1988 paper by Montreal physicians states that the treatments have severe side effects, such as peripheral neuropathy, cytopenias and immune-system suppression.   A woman

72

who'd been treated with an anticancer drug, a steroid, colchicine, azathioprine [immune suppressant] and spleen removal required an emergency hysterectomy to prevent fatal loss of blood.

Four months after this trauma the woman began to take 2 grams of C a day. About a month later she noticed improvement in the little bleeding areas in her skin. Three months later her platelet count began to increase. At month 10 the count was normal. When physicians had her discontinue C the count declined, at a rate that would have dropped it to the previous low in about 3 months. A resumption of C intake returned her platelet count to its previous peak.

The physicians then gave 2 grams of C every morning to 11 adults with ITP. Seven were "complete responders" in that C kept the platelet count in the normal range. Platelet count in two others rose somewhat but declined later [probably because of the tolerance effect]. And C was considered to be ineffective in the the remaining two, although the count rose more than 25%.[10] Some patients doubled the dose, according to a letter the lead author wrote to another journal.[11] They must have sensed the need for more C.

The above report encouraged Japanese physicians to try C on a woman, 23, who'd already had her spleen removed and was on immune-suppressing drugs. No therapy had helped. On 2 grams of C a day her platelet count rose to normal in 4 months. The title of the English abstract says it all:

CHRONIC ITP WITH A REMARKABLE RESPONSE TO VITAMIN C ADMINISTRATION AFTER SPLENECTOMY.[12]

The fact that purpura is one of the signs of scurvy suggested to physicians years ago that extra C would be a logical treatment. In 1935 the urinary output of C registered far lower than normal in 5 purpuric patients. It also failed to rise significantly, as it does in normal individuals, when 100 mg were given intravenously, indicating a substantial need by the body.[13] Later studies found normal C levels in some purpuric patients and the results of 1-gram studies were inconclusive. Because C was not owned by a company that could profit from pursuing the leads, it failed to become an early treatment for the disease.

Following the Montreal and Japanese reports, the *British Journal of Haematology* published 6 reports from others who had tried C for ITP [1990; 74:234-5 and 75:623-7]. In Belgium only 1 of 14 patients improved markedly on the 2-gram dose. A trial in Britain with 2 grams ended in disappointing results also. In a Japanese report, the 2-gram dose caused platelet count to rise initially in all but one patient but then declined. The same low dose given to 8 patients in London followed the same pattern of rise and decline except in one whose count rose to normal and stabilized. A Kuwaiti woman with a stubborn 5-year case took a gram of C twice a day. Platelet count began to rise during the second week of treatment and was remaining at a satisfactory level when reported 8 weeks later. A 6-month trial in which 3 adults in northern England took half-gram tablets of C 4 times a day was judged a failure. As in some of the other studies, a rise in count occurred, then fell back or rose no further.

The lesson should be clear: In most cases a 2-gram daily dose is not enough.

A 1991 Italian report involved 9 children, ages 3 to 15. The inadequate and ineffective doses ranged from less than a gram to slightly more, depending on the size of the child.[14] Four of seven Israeli children in the same age range fared better on 500 mg of C given 3 times a day. The other three were not helped. The authors felt that C should be tried before other therapy.[15]

Another Italian ITP study involved 8 children, aged 4 to 16. Each took a single 2-gram dose every morning before breakfast. So large a dose on an empty stomach can speed through the gut of some individuals so quickly that absorption is minimal. Two children did absorb enough to be cured, however. The others failed to respond, according to the authors, but a table in the report shows platelet counts in 3 of them rose higher than in the two cured cases before falling back to a 10% to 20% gain.

As in the preceding studies, doses were not increased to compensate for tolerance. Even though the low dose achieved a 25% cure rate, the authors of the report felt that C was useless, concluding "...the results of this study, together with those reviewed in the literature, [do] not support the use of ascorbic acid in the treatment of chronic childhood ITP."[16]

We assume that all their future patients will be subjected to the full range of traumatic treatments for the disease. Bias is hard on patients. A hematologist wrote me that he has used C in the treatment of purpura for years. At a convention he was allowed to present a paper detailing his favorable experience---but could not get the information published in a medical journal.

Inadequate dosing is seen in nearly all reports on the use of extra C, even when the benefits are impressive [chapter 7]. In some cases, the use of higher amounts or more frequent administration would increase the benefit as well as the percentage of patients responding to treatment.

References

1   DeCosse J J, Adams M B, Kuzma J F, et al. Effect of ascorbic acid on rectal polyps of patients with familial polyposis. *Surgery* 1975; 78:608-12

2   Watne A L, Lai H Y, Carrier J, Coppula W. The diagnosis and surgical treatment of patients with Gardner's syndrome. *Surgery* 1977; 82:327-33

3   Bussey H J R, DeCosse J J, Deschner E E, et al. A randomized trial of ascorbic acid in polyposis coli. *Cancer* 1982; 50:1434-9

4   McKeown-Eyssen G, Holloway C, Jazmaji V, et al. A randomized trial of vitamins C and E in the prevention of recurrence of colorectal polyps. *Cancer Research* 1988; 48:4701-5

5   DeCosse j j, Miller H H, Lesser M L. Effect of wheat fiber and vitamins C and E on rectal polyps in patients with familial adenomatous polyposis. *J Natl Cancer Inst* 1989; 81:1290-7

6   Paganelli G M, Biasco G, Brandi G, et al. Effect of vitamin A, C, and E supplementation on rectal cell proliferation in patients with colorectal adenomas. *J Natl Cancer Inst* 1992; 84:47-51

7   Roncucci L, Di Donato P, Carati L, et al. Antioxidant vitamins or lactulose for the prevention of the recurrence of colorectal adenomas. *Dis Colon Rectum* 1993; 36:227-34

8   Spigelman A D, Uff C R, Phillips R K S. Virtamin C levels in patients with familial adenomatous polyposis. *Br J Surg* 1990; 77:508-9

9   Gasbarrini A, Franceschi F, Tartaglione R, et al. Regression of autoimmune thrombocytopenia after eradication of Helicobacter pylori. *Lancet* 1998; 352:878

10 Brox A G, Howson-Jan K, Fauser A A. Treatment of idiopathic thrombocytopenic purpura with ascorbate. *Br J Haematol* 1988; 70:341-4

11 Brox A. Ascorbate for the treatment of refractory idiopathic thrombocyto-penic purpura (letter). *Br J Haematol* 1990; 74:234-5

12 Nomura S, Yanabu M, Soga T, et al. Chronic ITP with a remarkable response to vitamin C administration after splenectomy. *Rinsho Ketsueki* 1990; 31:523-4

13 Finkle P. Observations on excretion of vitamin C in some vascular diseases. *Proc Soc Experi Biol Med* 1935; 32:1163-4

14 Ramenghi U, Saracco P, Timeus F, et al. Use of ascorbate for the treatment of refractory idiopathic thrombocytopenic purpura in children. *Am J Pediatric Hematol/oncol* 1991; 13:486-9

15 Cohen H A, Nussinovitch M, Gross S, et al. Treatment of chronic idiopathic thrombocytopenic purpura with ascorbate. *Clin Pediatrics* 1993; 32:300-02

16 Amendola G, Cirillo G, Spiezie M. et al. Treatment of childhood chronic idiopathic thrombocytopenic purpura with ascorbate. *Clin Pediatrics* 1995; 34:268-70

5

Side Effects, Real And Alleged; And Safety

At a certain level of higher intake C begins to act like a drug, therefore can be expected to cause side effects, as do other drugs. Probably the side effect that would bother the greatest number of the 20% who cannot tolerate much extra C is one of the nuisance reactions that occur upon taking a gram or two. An increase in intestinal gas heads the list. Gut cramps and/or loose stools are a close second. Some persons can avoid the problem by taking timed-release pills, although loose stools will occur if an overactive gut speeds them to the colon before they dissolve completely. Vitamin C is the perfect laxative when taken judiciously. External signs of distress from extra C appear in the form of blisters around the mouth or a light rash in other areas.

People taking anticoagulants ["blood thinners"] comprise the second greatest number of people who can have problems with extra C. Call it a drug interaction rather than a side effect if you wish. C diminishes the effectiveness of warfarin. It's quite logical that it should: warfarin is a diluted toxin---and C is antitoxic.

In 1971 a physician reported the case of a woman who was hospitalized with a blood clot in a lung. He injected heparin initially then stabilized her on warfarin. About a month after her hospital discharge the warfarin began to lose its effect. The dose was doubled, then almost tripled before becoming effective again. The doctor asked if she'd been taking other medication or eating food high in vitamin K, which promotes clotting. She said no. Further questioning revealed that she was taking extra C in the mornings to ward off colds. The amount was not stated. Her warfarin requirement returned to the original dose 2 days after she stopped taking extra C.[1]

Animal studies done earlier had shown that the effect is minimal when only a little C is taken. No need for extra warfarin occurred when 5 patients took a gram of C a day for 2 weeks[2] but it was necessary to increase the warfarin dose 5-fold when a 70-year-old woman took 16 grams a day.[3]

A group of patients each took 3 grams of C a day for a week, then 5 grams a day during the second week. The warfarin dose remained stable, as it did in those who took 10 grams a day for a week. However, the blood level of the anticoagulant was reduced by as much as 40% [mean17.5%][4], suggesting that the results of a short-term study may be misleading. A longer period on high-dose C might lower the anticoagulant level even more. People on anticoagulant should monitor its response to extra C.

Another drug interaction involves estrogen. Contraceptive pills that contain it will lower plasma and white-cell C.[5,6] Some side effects of the pill may be due to the lower C levels. One investigator advised taking 500 mg of C a day to compensate.[7] Estrogen causes the liver to raise the blood level of ceruloplasmin, a copper compound that can destroy C. In addition, estrogen and C have their own interaction, as C is said to convert a low-dose pill into a high-dose one.[8]

As the use of C accelerated in the 1970s the list of possible side effects expanded in proportion. Some were legitimate concerns but others seemed to be, as Klenner wrote, scare weapons brandished by critics or special-interest groups. The word went out, for example, that extra C causes infertility. The folks in Ireland in the 1800s would have laughed at that one. In the years when potatoes supplied them with a gram of C a day the population of the island was more than *twice* what it is now. [Many Irish adults ate up to 14 **pounds** of potatoes a day,[9] which supplied a daily gram of C as a year-round average and 1.5 grams in fall, as new potatoes contain 50% more C.]

Once expressed, a baseless warning about C reverberates in the public mind for years. It may turn away a reasoning person as effectively as a black cat repels a superstitious one. A brief statement that an alleged side effect is unfounded may not be enough to dispel all the doubts about C in a reader's mind. He or she would be better served by a condensation of the literature on the subject in order to develop a better understanding---firm insights not likely to be jarred loose by the sort of scary tales told about black cats. So bear with us while we present the literature.

After Linus Pauling sparked public interest in C the opportunity arose for making a career in bashing it regularly. In 1974 a critic reported that a half gram of C destroyed up to 95% of vitamin B12 in a test meal that was kept at room temperature for a half hour.[10]   That's a big scary percentage to someone who isn't aware that even if 100% were destroyed, 3 or 4 years would pass before the average body would notice.   [An article in the February, 2000 issue of *Discover* states that a vegetarian without a dietary source of B12 remained in good health for 38 years before showing signs of deficiency.]

Old folks are apt to have low blood levels of B12. Their levels of C are usually low also, reason enough to investigate the claim that taking extra C would be hazardous. The controversy lasted for almost 10 years before the medical community was satisfied that C is no threat to our B12 status.

Physicians began to check patients who were taking extra C to acidify the urine. To a report that no deficiency of B12 was found, the critic replied that dietary iron may have protected it; or that the C may have been taken between meals; or that liver disease may have accounted for some of the higher readings; or that the physician's test for B12 may have been faulty.[11]

Other physicians reported that none of their patients on extra C had low B12 levels. Two independent laboratories found the B12 in the critic's test meal to be less than he had calculated, therefore the amount of destruction by C was overstated. It was concluded that "...there is no significant deleterious effect of added ascorbic acid on vitamin B12 stability in foods..."[12]

Still, opposite opinions kept the issue alive for several more years. Some experts straddled the issue for fear of being on the wrong side when it was settled. A number of test-tube studies were done, some not very practical at first glance, such as boiling C and B12 in blood serum. A first thought is that a guy being barbecued couldn't care less about his B12 status. But the effort yielded important chemical information. Resolution of the differences neared an end when sensitive test methods described in a 1980 report found no threat to the B12 level, even at C concentrations as high as 10 mg per milliliter,[13] about 100 times the normal level of C in the bloodstream.

A 1982 report finally ended the controversy. Ingested B12 was followed by radiotracer techniques through the body of both healthy persons and patients with pernicious anemia who were taking *intrinsic factor*, the substance they lack which is necessary for absorption of B12. It was seen that B12 binds so quickly and firmly to intrinsic factor that C could not destroy it.[14]

Thus a test meal---which was never in a stomach---created a bogie that medical textbooks continued to mention as a hazard up to 15 years after research had shown it to be a false alarm.

Another skirmish in the effort to label extra C a hazard, or at least a nuisance, heated up when a 1976 report stated that a single 4-gram dose increased the amount of urinary uric acid and might cause symptoms of gout.[15] The discomfort of gout is due to urate crystal deposits in the joints and elsewhere. It is linked with a high blood level of uric acid. Drugs taken to reduce this level increase the amount in urine. Gouty symptoms may appear when the drugs are first taken. The warning went out that large doses of C might also cause the symptoms as well as put gout-prone people at risk of developing urate kidney stones. Two other reports soon followed, confirming that extra C raised the blood level of uric acid.[16, 17]

Reports to the contrary then appeared, in which doses of 4, 8, 10, and 12 grams were used.[18, 19] Investigators reported in 1983 that test methods not specific for uric acid will result in false high readings.[20] The information made earlier reports unreliable. No case of gout flare-up or urate stones due to extra C turned up, so the concern soon faded, yet some recent editions of medical textbooks still mention that extra C increases the blood level of uric acid.

Uric acid is an antioxidant. Perhaps a small rise in its level would be desirable. It is said that gout and multiple sclerosis are "mutually exclusive," that is, a gout-prone person seldom contracts multiple sclerosis, and vice versa. Some trivia: besides humans and their primate cousins, the only other animal known to form urate kidney stones is the Dalmatian dog.

It is not the urate stone that alarmists have in mind when extra C is mentioned. It is the oxalate stone. A percentage of the C ingested, whether as food or supplement, converts to oxalate in the body. Most stones are of the oxalate type, therefore most of the concern about taking extra C is focused on oxalate stones.

Like all excursions into the realm of the possible, each re-printing leans more toward the probable until eventually the slim chance is presented as a sure thing. But there's no scientific evidence to support the hypothesis. Although reports of an association between C and stones is seen in earlier literature, the hunting season on the vitamin opened in earnest after Pauling's first book on the common cold was published in 1970.

A 1972 paper mentioned C as a cause of stones but another physician argued that no stones occurred in patients during his many years of prescribing extra C. In reply, the author of the first paper wrote that C accounts for up to a third of the urinary oxalate; and although a high intake may add only a little more, it could increase the tendency to form stones.[21, 22] Now the hunt was on for hard evidence.

Among the conditions associated with stones are diseased bowels; removal of all or part of the upper intestine; errors in metabolism; vitamin B-6 deficiency; excess bile acid; low fluid intake; and excessive consumption of high-oxalate substances such as rhubarb, spinach, tea or cocoa. A "stone epidemic" that plagued British troops in India was attributed to excessive consumption of tea to make life bearable in the hot dry climate.

The terms oxalate and oxalic acid are often used interchangeably. Of the common food items, cocoa powder contains the highest percentage of oxalate at 623 mg per 100 grams. Except for chocolate addicts, it is not as significant a dietary source as spinach and rhubarb, which contain roughly 550 mg per 100 grams. Beetroots are the next highest source, with about 100 mg per 100 grams. Instant coffee contains very little oxalate per cup. Tea has 30 to 60 mg, depending on the strength.

The usual daily intake of oxalate is about 70 mg. Normally, about 5% is absorbed but those who form stones regularly appear to absorb more. Vitamin D appears to increase oxalate absorption, as does a low-calcium diet. Low vitamin B-6 promotes the build-up of a precursor to oxalate and also decreases the acidity of urine. A low level of magnesium reduces urinary citrate, which allows oxalate to precipitate out of solution.[23]

Researchers reported in 1980 that daily C intake of a gram and 6 grams did not increase urinary oxalate in either stone-formers or non-stone-formers. They noted that stone-formers have low levels of phosphate and citrate, substances that inhibit formation of oxalate crystals. A man under study had been on a beetroot diet. He was said to have ingested 500 mg of oxalate a day for 5 years. There were oxalate crystals in his urine---but he had no stones. The researchers felt that C is not a risk factor in stone formation.[24] C advocates would agree. Klenner wrote that urinary output must be low and neutral or alkaline before stones can form, and that extra C is both a diuretic and an acidifier [ref 14, chapter 1,].

But a stone expert wrote that oxalate can precipitate out of normal acidic urine. And that 4 or more grams of C a day taken for a year or more might be enough to cause stones in persons who form them regularly. He cited 5 cases: each individual had taken at least 4 grams of C a day. Each developed a stone from 1 to 3 years afterward.[25]

The account is anecdotal evidence, you know. The type that would be sniffed at if a doctor reported that 4 grams of C a day aborted colds in 5 patients. Doubters could argue that a patient who developed a stone after 3 years on extra C should have been free of stones for 3 years prior to the start of the C regimen to be sure that a stone wouldn't occur every 3 years anyway. And confirmation would require another 6 years of observation. [You need a trial lawyer's mind to compete in that league.]

The method of handling a urine specimen and measuring its oxalate caused many of the false highs in early studies that associated C with stones. Delaying analysis allows the C in a specimen to convert to oxalate. Its content can increase 4-fold if a specimen is left overnight at room temperature.[26] There are reports that C given intravenously has resulted in blockage of kidney tubules with oxalate.[27,28,29] The solutions may not have been fresh, so that oxalate rather than C was given. This is not a concern anymore; trained therapists use fresh solutions.

One of the reasons critics say that taking large amounts of C is useless is that studies have shown the body can't utilize it because the absorption rate tapers off dramatically after 2 to 3 grams are absorbed. Taking this and other factors into account, chemists calculated that a 155-pound man would need to take 36 grams a day to be in the range where a stone might occur.[26]

People who form stones regularly handle C differently. They convert most of the ingested C to oxalate *in the gut*, then absorb the oxalate. It's as if they were living on spinach and rhubarb. This of course leads to stones if conditions are right. If most of it converts to oxalate, do stone-formers have enough C left to keep its blood level up? No. Regular stone-formers have low C levels, either due to oxalate conversion or malabsorption. When a group of stone-formers were given 500 mg of C intravenously they failed to pass the expected amount in the urine. The body needed it, therefore refused to give it up.[30]

Of the dozens of studies on oxalate, This effort appears to have measured it with the greatest accuracy: Urine from one kidney of each participant went via tube directly to a collection pouch in which a preservative immediately blocked any change in C or oxalate status. The other kidney drained into the bladder, then by catheter into a pouch. When each pouch contained the preservative, no difference was seen. But up to 32% more oxalate was found in specimens that lacked the preservative when 100 and 500 mg of C were taken, with a comparable reduction in C because of its conversion to oxalate. Doses of 1,000 and 2,000 mg almost doubled the percentage of error.[31]

The final stake in the heart of the kidney-stone bogie came with the analysis of data gathered from questionnaires about the diertary habits of healthcare professionals---the ongoing Harvard Study. After excluding those who'd already had stones, the diet and vitamin intake of 45,251 men were checked for a linkage between C and stones, and vitamin B-6 and stones.   Over a 6-year period, 751 men developed stones. A check of their diets revealed that *the C intake of those who developed stones was significantly* **lower** *than intake by those who had not developed stones!* Conclusion: "Our findings provide no support for the belief that intake of even high doses of vitamin C or B6 is associated with the formation of kidney stones."[32]

When the aminoquinoline drugs like primaquine came into use for treating malaria they caused a substantial destruction of red blood cells in a few patients. Viral infections and a long list of common drugs such as sulfas and phenacetin also destroy red cells in those few.

And so does extra C. The red cells of the affected people have low levels of the enzyme glucose-6-phosphate dehydrogen-ase [G6PD]. Of interest is that this condition which renders them vulnerable to modern medicines confers more resistance to the ancient scourge, falciparum malaria. A shortage of the enzyme restricts parasite numbers, resulting in a milder disease.

A small percentage of people in the U.S. who have genetic roots in Africa, around the Mediterranean and eastward to southern China have low amounts of G6PD. Roughly ten times more men than women are affected. About 11% of African American men, 6% of men in southern China and 3% of Taiwanese men have varying degrees of low G6PD. There are many different types. One type causes favism, a sensitivity to fava beans, which is more common around the Mediterranean, especially in Italy. Eating the beans or even inhaling the pollen from its flowers can cause massive red-cell destruction in some individuals.

Only mild destruction occurred when 1.5 grams of C were taken by volunteers who were severely deficient in the enzyme[33] but higher doses and intravenous administration can be fatal. A man with second-degree burns on his hand was given 80 grams of C intravenously on the first day of treatment and 80 more the next day. His urine turned brown with pigment from destroyed red cells on day three. His kidneys became clogged with debris and shut down. Other organs were affected also. In spite of intensive care, he died.[34]

An emergency case at a London hospital involved a man with low G6PD whose parents were Nigerian. A nutritionist had prescribed vitamins, fatty acids and glutathione plus 40 grams of C intravenously 3 times a week along with 20 to 40 grams of C orally. The treatment continued for a month with no ill effect. [It gives you an idea how much C a sick man can take. He had AIDS.]

Then the intravenous dose was increased to 80 grams. Next day the man's urine turned black, his breathing became labored and his temperature rose. Two days later he was hospitalized. Treatment consisted of giving folic acid, amount not stated, and 4 to 5 liters of fluid a day orally. The blood pigments were flushed out by day 3 of the hospital stay and he was discharged on day 4. It was thought that glutathione had prevented destruction of red cells by the 40-gram intravenous doses of C but could not do so when 80 grams were given.[35]

Another explanation might be that the 40-gram dose was being used up in treating the viral infection, leaving none to destroy red cells. We can speculate that the destruction would not have occurred if the intravenous dose had been increased gradually until the highest useful amount had been reached.

In India, a boy, 10, who had passed "cola colored" urine for a day became increasingly distressed so that he required hospitalization. A day later his cousin developed a similar but milder case. Over a period of about 6 hours they had drank several imitation orange drinks that contained about 75 mg of C per glass, plus 2 or 3 glasses of a lemon drink containing a gram of C per glass---a total of about 4 grams each. Not much, normally, but the boys had low G6PD, as did their mothers.[36]

A suggested do-it-yourself screening for low G6PD involves increasing C intake by a gram every third day while observing the color of the urine.

Individuals who have genetic roots in areas where low G6PD is common but are not extremely deficient themselves may think they have no reason to be concerned. But if they plan to raise a family they should be warned that their children could inherit a severe deficiency. A Chinese baby in California died of massive red-cell destruction two hours after being born. To ease a cold the mother had taken up to 500 mg of C a day for 2 weeks before delivery. She had eaten a few fava beans also. Her roots were in southern China where favism occurs. The small amount of extra C may not have been the major factor in the baby's death.[37]

But just in case, if low G6PD is suspected, the mother should limit C intake to the RDA. Destruction of red cells in the baby may not be lethal but the excess billirubin that results, if severe enough, could lead to complications. A study of a group of African-American newborns ruled out every possible cause of hyperbillirubinemia except low G6PD in combination with high blood levels of C in the babies.[38]

Individuals with sickle-cell anemia can be distressed by extra C. A substantial percentage have low G6PD also.[39]   This rare type of anemia afflicts Blacks almost exclusively. In the U.S. about one in ten carries the trait [gene]. One in 400 inherits the disease. A woman with the disease had a typical sickle-cell "crisis" whenever she took extra C for a cold.[40]

Still another rare blood disease, paroxysmal nocturnal hemo-globinuria [PNH], has been triggered by extra C. This type of red-cell destruction occurred after a Japanese man, 24, drank large quantities of a soft drink that was enriched with more than 2 grams of C per cup. He and two other individuals with PNH experienced the same reaction after drinking C-enriched tea, a popular beverage in Japan.[41]

Long-term consumption of food or drink having excessive amounts of iron can lead to a condition similar to hereditary iron-overload diseases such as hemochromatosis. In the 1920s, autopsies revealed excessive iron deposits in the bodies of Bantu men and women in South Africa. Physicians became more interested in the 1950s. Since then dozens of studies have been reported.

The livers of 20% of men who died in a Johannesburg hospital contained as much iron as is found in the livers of patients with hereditary hemochromatosis. This was first attributed to iron leaching from pots in which food was cooked. But the condition afflicted more men than women, leading to a suspicion that the home-brewed beer fermented in big iron kettles or steel oil drums was loaded with iron. It was---about 9 mg per cup. The amount could be as high as 750 times that found in commercial beer produced in the United States.[42]

The body regulates its iron absorption very well when food and drink contain a normal 15 to 25 mg a day but the food and beer consumed by the Bantu supplied from 35 to 215 mg of iron a day. Iron slowly accumulated in the tissues. Some of the men had scurvy, leading to the observation that excess iron destroys C; that a low level of C occurs in all cases of iron overload.

The low level is thought to be caused by two factors. First, iron that accumulates in the cells lining the intestinal wall destroy C in the process of being absorbed. Second, the C that manages to get past this hazard is destroyed by excess iron in other tissues. Much of the C in this last reaction is converted to oxalic acid, more than doubling the normal rate of oxalate excretion. Iron-overloaded individuals excreted about 4 times more oxalate than normals when 250 mg of C were injected intramuscularly every 8 hours. Because of its conversion to oxalate, the amount of C excreted was proportionately less.[43]

Researchers suspected that a gene-linked susceptibility is involved in this type of iron overload because not all beer drinkers develop it, even though the iron content in a liter of their beer was 80 mg. Several liters a day were downed on weekends. A study of the members of 36 families in Zimbabwe confirmed the gene hypothesis. Those who had the gene were overloaded.[44] Its prevalence in the world population is not known.

Iron overload in patients with hereditary anemias such as thalassemia is due to the many transfusions received. It has been suggested that they might be better off with a low level of C in order to limit its destructive reaction with iron in the tissues.[45] Iron and C have both a beneficial and detrimental relationship. C is used as an aid to absorption of iron and also in chelation tharapy to remove an excess. But heart function will deteriorate if too much C is given. Only 500 mg damaged the hearts of 8 patients in a group of 11 undergoing chelation therapy. Luckily, heart function improved in 6 after C was discontinued.[46] It may have improved in the other 2 later, as recovery can be slow.

A slow recovery was seen in a man who was anemic due to a deficiency of the enzyme pyruvate kinase in his red cells. He was thought to have become overloaded with iron because of excessive intestinal absorption since he'd had only one transfusion during a surgery. However, he had taken iron tablets for a few months without realizing he didn't need them. For 3 years during the overloaded condition, he had taken a half gram of C a day without a problem but 9 months after raising the daily dose to a gram he began to tire quickly during exercise. His heart was failing. The C regimen was discontinued and iron-removal therapy begun. Heart function did not improve noticeably until 17 months had passed.[47, 48]

More rapid heart damage and quicker recovery occurred when a man, overloaded with iron due to many transfusions, began to take 4 grams of C a day. About a month later his heart was failing. Ejection fraction, a measure of function, reached a low of 20% [normal range: 57-73%]. Eight months after the start of chelation therapy the ejection fraction had increased to 50%.[49]

Most of us are not overloaded with iron but anyone who has had many transfusions or has relatives with overload should know his or her iron status before beginning a long-term C regimen of more than 500 mg a day. Although the condition is rare, a person can have a subclinical form of hemochromatosis without knowing it. In such a case, taking extra C would be harmful.

A 1982 report should alert everyone to the risk: At age 29 an Australian man, in good enough health to play competition rugby football, began to feel tired about a month after a recent game. Two months later he was hospitalized with debilitating fatigue and shortness of breath. He had been taking a gram of C a day plus an unstated amount of artificial orange juice.

The clinical signs were those of heart failure. His heart was enlarged and loaded with iron, as were the liver, pancreas and lymph nodes. Yet his serum iron content was in the normal range, pointing out that the test is unreliable as an indicator of iron overload. Only the high readings of ferritin and transferrin saturation confirmed the diagnosis. In spite of intensive care, he died. Two of his six siblings were seen to have subclinical hemochromatosis also. They were not aware of it.[50]

Occasionally we hear it said that no one has ever died from taking too much vitamin C. Certainly the event is rare but it can happen---in cases of iron overload, low G6PD and PNH.

Tolerance of extra C, sometimes termed *tachyphylaxis*, leads to a dependence that is termed *systemic conditioning*. Tolerance was mentioned in earlier chapters. In his 1974 report [chapter 2], Anderson expressed concern about "the rapidity with which abnormally low blood levels of ascorbic acid develop following the abrupt withdrawal of a high daily dose." He felt it might be detrimental if it coincided with acute illness or need for surgery. In 1975 he referred to it as "the indirect hazard of dependency."

Cathcart wrote of it in 1981, of its being more noticeable at doses above 4 grams a day. He advised that high dosers carry a wallet card to alert hospital personnel in case of emergency. With luck, the high dose would then be continued. Ideally it would be increased to supply the extra needs of a stressed body. The ideal is seldom achieved, though, either because of bias or the belief that conditioning doesn't occur. An expert found no convincing evidence in healthy individuals in the literature---no scientific proof, therefore it didn't exist. [If we relied exclusively on scientific proof we'd be in trouble. No human trial has proved that certain mushrooms are poisonous, for example.]

Since people who take high doses are presumed to be a bit daft, perhaps they qualify as being unhealthy, thereby protecting the expert from the barbs of others who knew he was wrong. Discontinuing a *long-term* high dose can cause upsets that range from scurvy to a listless weariness the lasts for days unless the high dose is resumed.

A woman stopped a high dose for a few weeks while on a trip. She developed the swollen legs that are sometimes seen in scurvy. The swelling didn't resolve until after she resumed the high dose [personal observation]. A man drank many glasses of orange juice while working in the Florida groves. After he quit and returned to Sweden he developed scurvy. The term *rebound scurvy* is used in reference to a reaction this severe. When the supply of C ran out during the siege of Leningrad in World War II, citizens who had been taking higher amounts developed scurvy sooner than those who had not taken supplements.[51]

You'll recall that the Irish enjoyed a high C diet before the potato shortage [page 77]. Due to the drastic reduction of their C intake, more of them died from scurvy and other diseases than from starvation. And we saw that terminal cancer patients who had been abruptly deprived of high-dose C died sooner than those on placebo [page53]. A baby whose mother had taken large doses of C during pregnancy could be at risk of developing scurvy soon after birth.[52] It should be given extra C that would be tapered down to optimal intake after a time.

There's a wide range of individual difference with respect to conditioning/tolerance. Young resilient persons may not even notice a drastic reduction in C intake but those of middle age and up will not fare as well. Anyone in that age bracket who doubts the existence of this feature of C needn't wait on a scientific trial for proof. A veteran of high-dose C advises taking 10 grams a day for a month, then stopping abruptly. Listlessness is the minimum result. The maximum, or close to it, are the aches that result from being galloped over by a stampede. The older one is, the greater the phantom hoofprint count.

In this chapter we've seen that extra C, contrary to what its most avid critics had claimed, is not a horribly toxic substance that we should never consume. Most of the warnings expressed in the 1970s and 1980s were shown to be ghost stories.

But the effort to hammer it back into medical limbo never lets up. An article in *Nature*, April 9, 1998, created much ado about the pro-oxidant properties of C and how it would damage our DNA. Researchers have known of the property for years. It is said to be the reason for its antiviral activity. Other sub-substances---wine, for example, which is promoted as beneficial to the cardiovascular system---contains pro-oxidants also. perhaps C was singled out because of the need to scare the populace away from it again. The old kidney-stone bugaboo isn't working anymore.

According to the article, 30 people took 500 mg of C a day for

6 weeks. The DNA in their lymphocytes was then shown to have oxidative damage, as determined by the increased amount of 8-oxoadenine and a decreased amount of 8-oxoguanine. Those substances were said to be markers [indicators] for DNA damage due to oxygen radicals.

Authors of the paper warned that taking more than 500 mg a day might damage our DNA. Less C than that was said to be harmless, however, because the antioxidant effect predominates at lower doses. The *New York Times* quoted an author as saying that in view of their findings it would be unethical to test higher levels. It appeared to be a ludicrous attempt to limit research.

Veteran C experts didn't buy the study's conclusions. One said there were 10 things wrong with the study, that damage to DNA may have been done by the method used to test for it. Dr. Balz Frei, Director of the Pauling Institute at Oregon State University, agreed that 8-oxoguanine is indeed a marker for DNA damage---but it *decreased*, suggesting a protective effect of C. As for 8-oxoadenine, it is not an established marker for DNA damage. Even if it were, it is much less important than 8-oxoguanine. A later communication noted that 38 different human and animal studies had found that extra C *reduced* the number of markers that indicate damage to DNA.

Alan Woodall and Bruce Ames, in chapter 11 of *Vitamin C in Health and Disease*, edited by L Packer and J Fuchs [1997; Marcel Dekker, New york], stated that sperm cells "are unusually prone to oxidative damage," there being no "histone proteins or active DNA repair enzymes" which could protect against the damage. The seminal fluid, however, is loaded with C---8 times the concentration seen in blood plasma.

Mother Nature would be extremely foolish to concentrate C in seminal fluid if it was a threat to DNA! Studies have shown that damage is greater when the C level in seminal fluid is low! The corpus luteum that forms after ovulation is also loaded with C, as is follicular fluid. Instead being a threat to DNA, C stands guard all the way from the factory to point of delivery in order to protect the cargo from damage before conception! Experts who try to discredit C know this, of course. They just hope that news reporters and the general public will never catch on.

The heavy concentration of the vitamin in this important area doesn't deter critics from continuing to search for something harmful about extra C. Keep in mind there's a lot of money at stake. A paper in the June 15, 2001 edition of *Science* reported that C produces a substance that damages DNA. It's a test-tube study with no relation to conditions in living tissue. Test-tube studies are dismissed as artificial when C is shown to be of value but are well publicized when something against it turns up, such as the claim, from a test-tube study, that C destroys B12.

We shouldn't throw away the pills whenever news items report on what appears to be a downside of extra C. Those are man-bites-dog stories, the kind media folks are always looking for. The author of a 1995 review of the literature on the safety of antioxidants states there's no evidence that vitamin C induces damage to DNA in living beings.[53]

The authors of a 1996 paper on the safety of antioxidant vitamins concluded that, except for crystals and rare stones in patients with poor kidneys, C has no important adverse effects at doses less than 4 grams a day, but that it does interfere with certain laboratory tests.[54] [Data on higher doses is scarce.]

Some of the tests have been replaced with newer methods that are not affected by extra C. Nevertheless, patients should keep their doctors informed of their daily dose. To prevent distortion of blood or urine tests, extra-C intake should be stopped for a time before such tests are scheduled. The urinary excretion of a 10-gram daily dose taken for 2 weeks remained higher than normal for 2 days after it was stopped abruptly,[55] suggesting that high C intake should be discontinued for that long in order to ensure accurate test results. The time needn't be as long when testing stools for occult blood. Following the directions on the packet leaves time enough for C in the gut to clear---but it might be wise to avoid timed-release pills prior to sampling.

The safety record of C is better than that of any other medication. To put the issue in perspective a look in the *Abridged Index Medicus* is enlightening. That monthly publication's stated purpose is "to afford rapid access to selected biomedical journal literature of immediate interest to the practicing physician." Among the several sections that describe a medication's characteristics and uses is one titled *adverse effects.*

During the decade of the 1980s, the number of entries in the adverse-effects section under aspirin total 199. For all the penicillins, which are controlled by prescription and subject to more judicious use, the total is 88. The total for C is 14, during a decade when the hunting season on it was wide open. It is not a precise gauge but 14 is far short of aspirin's 199. Of the 14 for C, most were letters arguing about stones. One reported esophageal irritation from an acid tablet the didn't reach the stomach.

The image of C is slowly improving. Eliminating the term *megadose* would help. It suggests something monstrous. It was once said to be 10 times the RDA but has been used in reference to much higher doses, therefore has lost its meaning. An understanding of the amount in a *high dose* would help also. Researchers in a university setting may use the term in reference to a gram or two. Practicing physicians who treat with up to 200 grams a day would have a different idea of how high is high. Their experience comes from the response of hundreds of sick patients who are given doses beyond the amount said not to be absorbable, according to research. But remember: most research is done on healthy individuals who have no need for extra C.

In summary, it can be said that critics of C have greatly exaggerated the prevalence of its side effects while advocates have minimized them, particularly with respect to iron. Although millions of us are not at risk, thousands are probably ingesting more dietary iron or needlessly taking iron pills and bordering on overload. For them, dosing with more than a half-gram of C a day for more than a week could be detrimental.

Chapter 5 references

1 Rosenthal G. Interaction of ascorbic acid and warfarin.
   JAMA 1971; 215:1671

2 Hume R, Johnstone J M S, Weyers E. Interaction of ascorbic acid and warfarin. *JAMA* 1972; 219:1479

3 Smith E C, Skalski R J, Johnson G C, Rossi G V. Interaction of ascorbic acid and warfarin. *JAMA* 1972; 221:1166

4 Feetam C L, Leach R H, Meynell M J. Lack of a clinically important interaction between warfarin and ascorbic acid.
   Toxicol Appl Pharmacol 1975; 31:544-7

5 Rivers J M. Oral contraceptives and ascorbic acid.
   Am J Clin Nutr 1975; 28:550-4

6 Briggs M, Briggs M. Vitamin C requirements and oral contraceptives.
   Nature 1972; 238:277

7 Wynn V. Vitamins and oral contraceptive use. *Lancet* 1975 (1); 561-4

8 Briggs M H. Megadose vitamin C and metabolic effects of the pill.
   Br Med J 1981; 283:1547

9 Daly D C. The leaf that launched a thousand ships. *Natural History* 1996, January, pp24-32. And: *The Great Hunger*. Cecil Woodham Smith 1962. Harper & Row, New York

10 Herbert V, Jacob E. Destruction of vitamin B12 by ascorbic acid.
   JAMA 1974; 230:241-2

11 Afroz M, Bhothinard B, Etzkorn J R, et al. Vitamins C and B12.
   (letter and reply) Herbert V, Jacob E. *JAMA* 1975; 232:246

12 Newmark H L, Scheiner J, Marcus M, Prabhudesai M. Stability of vitamin B12 in the presence of ascorbic acid. *Am J Clin Nutr* 1976; 29:645-9

13 Marcus M, Prabhudesai M, Wassef S. Stability of vitamin B12 in the presence of ascorbic acid in food and serum: restoration by cyanide of apparent loss. *Am J Clin Nutr* 1980; 33:137-43

14 Watson W S, Vallance B D, Muir M M, Hume R. The effect of megadose ascorbic acid ingestion on the absorption and retention of vitamin B12 in man. *Scott Med J* 1982; 27:240-3

15 Stein H B, Hasan A, Fox I H. Ascorbic acid-induced uricosuria.
   A consequence of megavitamin therapy. *Ann Intern Med* 1976; 84:385-8

16 Del Arbol J L. Ascorbic acid and uricosuria. *Ann Intern Med* 1976; 85:829

17 Berger L, Gerson C D, Yu T F. The effect of ascorbic acid on uric acid excretion with a commentary on the renal handling of ascorbic acid.
   Am J Med 1977; 62:71-6

18 Schmidt K H, Hagmaier V, Hornig D H, Vuilleumier J P. Urinary oxalate excretion after large intakes of ascorbic acid in man.
   Am J Clin Nutr 1981; 34:305-11

19 Mitch W E, Johnson M W, Kirshenbaum J M, Lopez R E. Effect of large oral doses of ascorbic acid on uric acid excretion by normal subjects.
   Clin Pharmacol Ther 1981; 29:318-21

20 Fituri N, Allawi N, Bentley M, Costello J. Urinary and plasma oxalate during ingestion of pure ascorbic acid: a re-evaluation. *Eur Urol* 1983; 9:312-15

21 Smith L H, Fromm H, Hofmann A F. Acquired hyperoxaluria, nephrolithiasis and intestinal disease. *N Engl J Med* 1972; 286:1371-5

References

22   Poser E. Large ascorbic acid intake. (letter and reply)
     Smith, L H. *N Engl J Med* 1972; 287:412-13
23   Hagler L, Herman R H. Oxalate Metabolism. II
     Am J Clin Nutr 1973; 26:882-9
24   Butz M, Hoffmann H, Kohlbecker G. Dietary influence on serum and urinary
     oxalate in healthy subjects and oxalate stone formers.
     Urol Int 1980; 35:309-15
25   Herbert V. Risk of oxalate stones from large doses of vitamin C. [letter]
     And: Smith L.H reply [letter] *N Engl J Med* 1978; 298: 856
26   Conyers R A J, Bais R, Rofe A M, et al. Ascorbic acid intake, renal
     function, and urinary oxalate excretion. *Aust NZ J Med* 1985; 15:353-5
27   McAllister C J, Scowden E B, Dewberry F L, Richman A. Renal failure
     secondary to massive infusion of vitamin C. *JAMA* 1984; 252:1684
28   Swartz R D, Wesley J R, Somermeyer G, Lau K. Hyperoxaluria and renal
     insufficiency due to ascorbic acid administration during total parenteral
     nutrition. *Ann Intern Med* 1984; 100:530-1
29   Lawton J M, Conway L T, Crosson J T, et al. Acute oxalate nephropathy
     after massive ascorbic acid administration.
     Arch Intern Med 1985; 145:950-1
30   Chalmers A H, Cowley D M, Brown J M. A possible etiological role for
     ascorbate in calculi formation. *Clin Chem* 1986; 32:333-6
31   Urivetsky M, Kessaris D. Smith A D. Ascorbic acid overdosing: a risk factor
     for calcium oxalate nephrolithiasis. *J Urol* 1992; 147:1215-18
32   Curhan G C, Willett W C, Rimm E B, Stampfer M J. Prospective study of
     the intake of vitamins C and B6, and the risk of kidney stones in man.
     J Urol 1996; 155:1847-51
33   Brewer G J, Tarlov A R, Alving A S. Standardization of procedures for the
     study of glucose-6-phosphate dehydrogenase.
     WHO Tech Report 1967; 366:27
34   Campbell G D Jr., Steinberg M H, Bower J D. Ascorbic acid-induced
     hemolysis in G-6-PD deficiency. *Ann Intern Med* 1975; 82:810
35   Rees D C, Kelsey H, Richards J D M. Acute haemolysis induced by high
     dose ascorbic acid in glucose-6-phosphate dehydrogenase deficiency.
     BMJ 1993; 306:841-2
36   Mehta J B, Singhal S B, Bhupatrai C M. Ascorbic acid-induced haemolysis
     in G-6-PD defiency. *Lancet* 1990; 336;944
37   Mentzer W C Jr., Collier E. Hydrops fetalis associated with erythrocyte
     G-6-PD and maternal ingestion of fava beans and ascorbic acid.
     J Pediat 1975; 86: 565-7
38   Karayalcin G, Acs H, Lanzkowsky P. G-6-PD deficiency and
     hyperbilirubinemia in black American full-term infants.
     N.Y. State J Med 1979; Jan. 22-4
39   Steinberg M H, Dreiling B J. Glucose-6-phosphate dehydrogenase
     deficiency in sickle-cell anemia. *Ann Intern Med* 1974; 80:217-20
40   Goldstein M L. High-dose ascorbic acid therapy. *JAMA* 1971; 216:332-3

Chapter 5 references

41 Iwamoto N. Kawaguchi T. Horikawa K. et al. Haemolysis induced by ascorbic acid in paroxysmal nocturnal haemoglobinemia. *Lancet* 1994; 343:357

42 Gordeuk V R. Boyd R D. Brittenham G M. Dietary iron overload persists in rural sub-saharan Africa. *Lancet* 1986; (1):1310-13

43 Lynch S R. Seftel H C. Torrance J D. et al. Accelerated oxidative catabolism of ascorbic acid in siderotic Bantu. *Am J Clin Nutr* 1967; 20:641-7

44 Gordeuk V. Mukiibi J. Hasstedt S J. et al. Iron overload in Africa. *N Engl J Med* 1992; 326:95-100

45 Cohen A. Cohen I J. Schwartz E. Scurvy and altered iron stores in thalassemia major. *N Engl J Med* 1981; 304:158-60

46 Neinhuis A. Benz E J. Propper R. et al. Thalassemia major: molecular and clinical aspects. *Ann Intern Med* 1979; 91:833-97

47 Rowbotham B. Roeser H P. Iron overload associated with congenital pyruvate kinase deficiency and high dose ascorbic acid ingestion. *Aust NZ J Med* 1984; 14:667-9

48 Bett J H N. Wilkinson R K. Boyle C M. Iron overload associated with congenital pyruvate kinase deficiency and high dose ascorbic acid ingestion. *Aust NZ J Med* 1985; 15:270

49 Pestell R G. Barr A L. Brand G. Vitamin C and congestive heart failure. *Med J Aust* 1987; 147:153-4

50 McLaran C J. Bett J H N. Nye J A. Halliday J W. Congestive cardiomyopathy and haemochromatosis---rapid progression possibly accelerated by excessive ingestion of ascorbic acid. *Aust NZ J Med* 1982; 12:187-8

51 Rhead W J. Schrauzer G N. Risks of long-term ascorbic acid overdosage. *Nutr Rev* 1971; 29:262-3

52 Cochrane W A. Overnutrition in prenatal and neonatal life. a problem? *Can Med A J* 1965; 93:893-9

53 Diplock A T. Safety of antioxidant vitamins and B-carotene. *Am J Clin Nutr* 1995; 62s:1510s-16s

54 Meyers D G. Maloley P A. Weeks D. Safety of antioxidant vitamins. *Arch Intern Med* 1996; 925-35

55 Tsao C S. Salimi S L. Evidence of rebound effect with ascorbic acid. *Med Hypoth* 1984; 13:303-10

6

C 101
The Fundamentals

We were born with a higher blood level of C than we'll ever have again normally. As a fetus we'd rob Mom to keep our own level high. To counter the stress of birth our level was twice its level a day later. Afterward, our level averaged a third higher than Mom's, although there's wide variation among individuals.[1]

C in the milk of 25 *well nourished* mothers ranged from 4.4 to 15.8 mg per 100 ml. The concentration had no relation to the intake of C. The babies of these mothers ingested from 330 to 1018 ml of milk a day. It was calculated that, when fed naturally, the C intake of babies ranged from 49 to 86 mg a day. Human milk had twice the C of formula milk.[2]

Breast-fed babies usually have higher C levels than those on formula.[3] So formula-fed babies are shorted on C from day one, as are those given another mother's milk. Less than 10% of C remains in pasteurized human milk by the time it is given to babies.[4] Mothers' C level after delivery was down in the pre-scurvy range, on average.[1,4] [It may be a factor in post-partum blues.] Human milk has 3 to 4 times more C than cow milk.[5]

The National Academy of Sciences in spring, 2000 put the RDA [their term is now *dietary reference intake*] for C in infant diet at 40 mg during the first 6 months and 50 mg for the next 6 months. This is an increase over the 1989 RDA of 30 and 35, respectively. The adult RDA for women is now 75 mg; for men, 90, up from 50 and 60. Pregnancy and lactation RDA over age 18 is 85 and 120, respectively. Smokers should add 35 mg.

Infantile scurvy, called *Barlow's disease* a century ago, was relatively common then, even in affluent areas. A Norwegian pediatrician who was studying the disease recognized the condition in guinea pigs, thus alerting scientists to a common inexpensive animal that, like humans, cannot make its own C. The discovery, published in 1907, facilitated the study of the substance, not yet named, that could cure and prevent scurvy.

The C level is the amount in blood plasma or serum. The terms *plasma* and *serum* are sometimes used interchangeably. They're both clear fluids, the liquid part of the blood. The difference is that serum lacks the components that cause blood to clot. Serum is the clear fluid that oozes from a clot, having left those components behind. Most books put the normal range of C in plasma or serum at 0.4 to 1.5 mg per 100 milliliters [100 cc], which is a tenth of a liter [dl]. Think of it as a scant half cup. Some sources put the low normal at 0.6 instead of 0.4. It has been dropped to 0.2 in the 17th edition of the *Merck Manual*. An early authority felt that levels less than 0.75 should be considered subnormal. Those who know C well would agree.

The international system [SI] states the C level as micromoles per liter rather than milligrams per deciliter. It may be more convenient in chemical calculations but it's easier to visualize mg/dl as a lump about the size of a sesame seed in a scant half cup of liquid. A milligram of C is equal to 5.68 micromoles, so multiplying a milligram per deciliter by 10 gives us 56.8 micromoles per liter. The normal range of 0.4 to 1.5 mg/dl becomes 23 to 85 micromoles per liter [µmol/L]. To convert the SI figure to mg/dl, multiply the SI figure by the reciprocal of 56.8.

The C level in whole blood is a little higher than the level in plasma because of the high concentration of C in white cells and platelets. Plasma and red cells, with about equal concentrations of C, contain more than 70% of the C in blood. White cells and platelets contain the rest. The concentration in those cells is higher than that in red cells and plasma. It varies with the type of cell. The normal amount of C in white cells ranges from 16 to 36 micrograms per hundred million cells but a count as high as 72 micrograms has been reported. [Try visualizing that!]

Researchers usually measure plasma C. It's easier. Measuring the amount of C in the white cells is another way of determining the body's C status. This more tedious method is more revealing. It indicates the degree of saturation of body tissues. Plasma C is merely a measure of the C in the bloodstream at the moment, although if the amount has been rather constant over several days it reflects the general condition of the body with respect to C. In financial terms, plasma C can be compared to cash on hand while white-cell and tissue C compare with net worth. The "net worth" or body pool of C ranges from 1.5 to 3 or more grams. This is also stated as around 20 to 50 mg of C per kilogram of body weight.

The white-cell C total usually includes platelet C also. It is the C in the so-called buffy layer of centrifuged blood. Different types of white cells have different concentrations of C. The monocytes have the greatest concentration---80 times more than is found in an equal weight of plasma. Platelets have half as much and granulocytes about a third as much.[6]

Body organs differ from each other in C concentration also. The pituitary and adrenal glands are the leaders, having 40 to 50 mg of C per 100 grams of tissue. The eye lens: 25 to 31. Corpus luteum aside, those 3 tissues are in a class by themselves, having 2 to 10 times more C per 100 grams than other tissues---and up to 100 times more than an equal weight of plasma.[7] Concentration in the corpus luteum ranges from 24 to 48 mg per 100 grams normally and from 42 to 148 during pregnancy.[1]

The adrenal glands are the main storage depot for C. Albert Szent-Gyorgyi, who first reported isolating pure C, obtained it from the adrenal glands of cattle. Its concentration in the glands is 3 times greater than in orange juice. The adrenals are not a plentiful source, however. He accumulated less than an ounce of C during a year of processing the glands from a slaughterhouse. He had obtained small amounts from cabbages and other vegetables but didn't find a good inexpensive source until he tried red peppers. Within a few weeks he had extracted pounds of C.[8]

When body tissues have all the C they can hold they're said to be saturated, probably a "desirable state" an authority felt. It hasn't been proved that saturation provides definite benefits but we note that animals able to make their own C are programmed to keep its level at the saturation point.[9] In order to remain saturated, animals make **more** whenever they are sick or stressed. The stress in lab rats was once measured by their C status.

Humans can't make C, therefore sickness or other stress depletes them of the vitamin. *Humans should do consciously what animals do automatically when sick or stressed---load the bloodstream with C to satisfy the urgent need.* And they probably should keep their C level at the saturation point in order to remain in good health.

Saturation is determined by taking extra C for several days while measuring the amount that passes in the urine. An unsaturated body will retain and store much of the extra C during the first few days, then more and more of the daily dose is excreted as the tissues "fill up." When the tissues have taken up all the C they can hold, they're saturated, and the amount of urinary C becomes constant, varying only a little from day to day.[10]

An intake of 100 mg of C for only a few days will saturate healthy young individuals. Old folks need much more over a longer period of time. One study used 700 mg a day for 3 weeks.[11] In another study, a gram a day failed to raise the white-cell C up to the young-adult level.[12]

The diet of 2 groups of people over age 65 was supplemented with extra C, 40 mg a day for one group and 80 for the other. The C level rose steadily toward the young-adult level, finally reaching it in 9 months. It remained in that range for only 4 months, then began to decline.[13] This suggests that in some situations many months may pass before tolerance, or another factor, causes an increased requirement for C.

No matter how much C is taken orally, the plasma level normally peaks at around 2 or 3 mg per deciliter in healthy persons. Ewan Cameron, the late cancer specialist, stated in a personal note that his patients on 10 grams a day had plasma levels ranging from 2 to 6.8 mg per deciliter. Most were in the lower part of the range. Those with higher levels appeared to benefit more, suggesting that giving as much as possible intravenously without a downside would be more effective that oral dosing.

A letter to the *New England Journal of Medicine* [1981; 304:1491] states that a man who took 15 grams a day to treat a leg infection had a level of 17 mg per deciliter. The figure is out of the ball park. Perhaps it was meant to be 1.7 mg.

The C level was measured in some of the cold studies. On 3 grams a day, the highest plasma level reported by Schwartz was 1.48 mg/dl. Coulehan reported 2.39 mg/dl to be the mean high C level in pooled whole blood of boys aged 6 to 10 who took a gram of C a day. The high had been 1.42 mg/dl before the trial. The high in the older boys who took 2 grams a day was *less*: 2.06, up from 1.25 before the trial. It appears that the drop in the blood level of C as we age begins early in life.

A little C is absorbed by the inner cheek and stomach wall but most is absorbed in the small intestine, "escorted" by sodium. When large doses are taken and the escort service is at capacity, C can also reach the bloodstream by diffusion.[14, 15] It uses the same "escort system" that glucose uses to get into cells, therefore an excess of blood sugar will hinder cell absorption of C.

About 35% more C is absorbed, and more is retained by tissues, when taken with a citrus extract containing a *large* amount of bioflavonoids.[16] But the tiny amount of bioflavonoids in tablets on store shelves increases absorption only a little. Oral C peaks in the bloodstream in 30 minutes to 3 hours, smaller doses peaking earlier. More is absorbed when taken after food, particularly fatty food, because it moves through the gut slower, allowing C to remain in the absorption area longer.[17] Compared with an equal amount in a standard pill, C in a timed release pill will peak in the bloodstream at a lower level but is available for absorption longer. Its half-life in the body is twice that of a standard pill, allowing C to be of more use to the body.[18]

As C is being absorbed, some is already being eliminated. The body uses some, stores some and eliminates the rest, mostly as unused ascorbic acid, dehydroascorbic acid, diketogulonic acid, threonic acid and oxalate. About 97% of the unused C and its breakdown products in the bloodstream leaves via the urine. Most of the rest leaves via the bowel. [Very little leaves in perspiration---about 0.03 mg per 100 ml under exercise conditions that would produce 5 to 8 liters of sweat a day.[19]] And very little leaves in the breath as carbon dioxide.

The amount of C passed in the urine does not necessarily provide a true picture of the body's C status. If diseased kidneys are not eliminating it in the usual manner its level in the plasma will be higher than should be expected. If normal kidneys pass little or no C, however, they reflect accurately the plasma level, which would be down in the scurvy range.

In healthy well nourished individuals, the 97% that leaves via the urine represents 60 to 80 percent of the C that was ingested. It appears not to have been utilized---but some may have participated in oxidation-reduction reactions before being eliminated in its original state. Studies on *healthy* persons indicate that oral ingestion of 100 mg of C a day would be adequate for 95% of the populace. Smokers would need 140 mg a day.[20, 21]

Four papers reported depletion studies on 9 healthy prisoners around 1970. [At the start, 12 men were enrolled but 1 dropped out and 2 others took off for parts unknown.] They were put on a no-C diet for up to 99 days. On average, their reserve---the body pool of C---was used up at a rate of 3% per day, ranging from a low of 2.2% to a high of 4.1%. The high user developed severe scurvy. All exhibited signs and symptoms of scurvy by day 99.

The typical signs and symptoms seen in these studies were fatigue; small pinhead hemorrhages [petechiae] in the skin, which was rough due to hardened tissue encircling hair follicles; joint pain; gum disease; bleeding in joints; water retention; emotional stress; and mild acne. In some, a rash appeared around hair follicles. Pinhead skin hemorrhages appeared first. They did not enlarge to become big purple blotches as seen in classical scurvy of long duration. In the short term a well nourished body except for C presents a somewhat different scurvy picture than that seen in classical cases in which other nutrients may be lacking also.

The signs of scurvy appeared when the body pool, 1.5 to 3 grams, had declined to about 300 mg. After resumption of C intake, none passed in the urine until the body pool had built up to 1.5 grams. It was seen that, when well nourished otherwise, some individuals can get along on very little C. Only 6.5 mg of C a day cured scurvy in one of the men. This caused the authors to feel that a large daily intake of C is not necessary.[22, 23, 24, 25]

With breakfast, a nonsmoking healthy man took a gram of C a day for 2 days; then 2, 3, and 4 grams daily for 2 days each. Finally, 5 grams a day were taken for 10 days. During the last 7 days the dose was radiolabeled. Urinary C determined the amount absorbed. The **amount** absorbed was greater as the dose increased but the **percent** decreased: 75% of the gram dose was absorbed; 44% of the 2-gram dose; and 39% of the 3-gram dose. Absorption of the 4- and 5-gram doses did not exceed that from 3 grams. So we see that at 3 grams a day the absorption machinery is at capacity.

From this study it was calculated that a healthy body cannot absorb more than 1160 mg in a 24-hour period. [Remember that the man was a nonsmoker, not sick, and may not have been representative of the human average.] About 2.8% of the radiolabeled C and byproducts left via the bowel. Substantially more left in the urine---but about 75% couldn't be accounted for.[26]

Where did it go? Some of course remained in the body for a time, stored in the tissues. C doesn't come and go like tourists. A percentage settles in as the body "rotates its stock." The normal half-life of C in the body ranges from 8 to 20 days but is much longer when very little C is ingested. The greater the amount ingested, the shorter the half-life. It was thought that some of the labeled carbon of the C molecule may have left via the bowel as part of methane molecules. In this study neither the breath nor the nether wind was checked for labeled byproducts.

Guinea pigs differ from humans in that most of their C byproduct leaves in the breath. Very little C in humans goes out this way---although in iron overload a substantial portion of *ingested* C that has decomposed *before absorption* is found in the breath. This happens to a smaller degree with high doses in normals. It does not happen to C given intravenously, however.[27, 28]

A 1996 report of a study on how the body handles C tells us how much effort and inconvenience is involved. Seven healthy men were hospitalized, some for as long as 6 months, subjected to many lab tests, fed a low-C diet to deplete them toward scurvy, subjected to more tests, then were given increasing doses of C, up to 2.5 grams a day, over a period of several weeks.

They gave blood 24 times after ingesting 15 mg of C on the first day of reprieve from the low-C diet. On the second day the 15 mg were given intravenously. Blood was drawn shortly before and 17 times afterward during the 9-hour study. Contrary to the findings of the previous studies that suggested humans do not need much C, data gathered from this study indicate that the RDA is far too low. Many authorities have thought so for years but the dawdling before it is raised to a recommended 200 mg has been going on just as long because of conflicting opinions.

The current RDA of 75 mg is about a third of the amount that will raise plasma C level to the optimum, which is reached when about 200 mg are taken. Increases from doses higher than 200 mg were less dramatic. A gram a day increased the level by only 16%; the increase from 2.5 grams was lower yet. *Healthy* young individuals do not require amounts that large. The white cells accumulated all they needed from 100 mg a day.[29]

After noting the C requirement of guinea pigs and monkeys, Pauling felt that humans should take 1.75 to 3.5 grams a day. It's good advice for aging folks but the above study suggests that the young and healthy can do well with less. One can surmise that when our ancestors---Lucy's kin or whoever---gradually began grubbing for roots instead of picking fruits, those who couldn't stand the low-C diet perished early, done in either by illness or a stronger more efficient user of C who then passed on his genes. If humans can extract Chihuahuas and Saint Bernards from the genes in wolves and wild dogs, certainly Nature can create the conditions that produce humans who thrive on smaller amounts of C. The diet of hunter-gatherers supplied about 400 mg of C a day,[30] allowing them to thrive and populate the planet.

Even so the C-wasting genes are not bred out completely. Some individuals, and the sick and elderly who never made the scene during the stone age, do need much more C.

As mentioned, bioflavonoids aid in the absorption and utilization of C. [More is also absorbed from a C solution that is sipped slowly but the acid form will etch tooth enamel. Long-term use of the method is not advised.] Bioflavonoids are flavonoids the body can use. The trend is toward omitting "bio" and just calling them flavonoids. Some are powerful antioxidants. Some help prevent heart disease.[31] Some were once called vitamin P but the term was considered inappropriate by 1950.

Plants differ in the type of flavonoid produced. Vitamin C extracted from plants in the 1930s contained about 2.5% impurities, probably including flavonoids. The impure C was more than twice as effective as synthetic C in preventing paralysis and death of monkeys infected with poliomyelitis.[32] The early belief that natural C is better than the synthetic product probably stemmed from that report. We can return our C to the "impure" state by taking it with added flavonoids or with fruits and vegetables. Citrus flavonoids appear to work well with C.

Consider this 1937 report by two physicians, one a professor, at a university clinic in Copenhagen: Before synthetic C was available they cured scurvy with the juice of 5 to 10 lemons a day for a week or more. They switched to synthetic C after it became plentiful, giving 300 mg a day, the amount in the juice of 10 lemons. The synthetic C readily cured 26 of 29 patients---but had no effect on the other 3, *not even when given intravenously!* The 300 mg of injected C, equal to 600 mg of oral C, was in the bloodstream, available to the body but of no value because it could not be utilized. It even failed to raise the plasma C to normal. To achieve a cure it was necessary to give the patients lemon juice.[33] A look at the case histories of the 3 patients is of interest:

Case 1: A man, 24, had a history of diarrhea since age 7 and periods of ulcerative colitis since age 11 which improved in summer and fall when he ate fresh fruit and vegetables. All his teeth had been extracted. He bruised easily. At the start of treatment for scurvy his serum C was 0.02 to 0.03 mg per 100 ml. You'll recall that low normal is 0.4, more than 10 times the level found in this patient.

Oral doses of synthetic C, 300 mg a day for 10 days, failed to raise the level; nor did the same dose given intravenously for a few days. The juice of 5 lemons a day for 3 days raised it to 0.04. Doubling the lemon juice boosted the level to 0.2 on the first day, still below normal but out of the severe scurvy range. After 3 more days on the juice of 10 lemons a day, C began to appear in the urine. At day 7 serum C level was 0.26 but rising so that 5 lemons a day supplied C for the next 16 days, during which time serum C level reached a peak of 0.84 mg/dl and the scurvy vanished.

Case 2: For 15 years a man, 55, had experienced "hunger pain" and periods of gum disease. When seen in the clinic his stools were black due to bleeding in the gut. His serum C of 0.02 to 0.03 remained steady during 5 days of observation. 300 mg of synthetic C raised the level to 0.04. No C appeared in the urine. The same dose given intravenously raised the serum C level to 0.08 while 40 to 180 mg of C per day passed in the urine.

A switch to the juice of 10 lemons a day raised the C level to 0.69. Urinary C, which had not risen above 40 mg a day during the first 10 days jumped to 96 mg on day 11, indicating that the body could spare more. Notice that urinary C from injection of the synthetic product was much greater, probably because the body couldn't use it, therefore dumped it.

Case 3:   A woman, 44, had experienced stomach and intestinal trouble for 12 years---dyspepsia, diarrhea, colitis and bloody stools. During a 5-day observation period her serum C varied from 0.02 to 0.025 mg/dl. Ten days of oral synthetic C failed to raise it. Urinary C was zero. Ten days of intravenous synthetic C raised serum C to 0.08, the same amount seen in case 2. The urinary output was identical also---40 to 180 mg a day. During the next 6 days she drank the juice of 52 lemons, about 9 a day, which raised serum C to 66 mg/dl. Its urinary output rose from zero at start to 36 mg on day 5; and 82 on day 6, a signal that the dose was adequate.

The physicians noted the features these 3 patients had in common: an inability to absorb synthetic C or to utilize it when given intravenously; a response to lemon juice; and intestinal trouble of long duration. The lemon juice cured "both humoral and clinical abnormalities," which is to say that it restored serum C to normal and the diseased intestines to health. It appears that subclinical scurvy had targeted the intestines to cause discomfort for years before recognizable scurvy appeared.   The most unusual feature is of course the inability to utilize C.

If people having this rare condition existed in 1937, then wouldn't similar individuals exist today? Who are they? People who have tried all sorts of treatment without success? They may or may not be those with irritable-bowel syndrome, which some- times responds to antibiotic therapy. But it would be interesting to know the plasma C level in the stubborn cases.

The signs of scurvy do not always appear in the usual manner. Gum disease is often mentioned as a first sign but it may be just the most obvious sign. Capillary breakdown is a common early sign that results in pinhead hemorrhages in the skin. They may not be noticeable unless one is looking for them. About 30% of the populace is said to be deficient in C---but not so deficient that frank scurvy appears. In the days when scurvy was seen reg- ularly, physicians noticed that common illnesses often preceded it. They called the condition *subclinical scurvy*. Another appropriate term would be *target-organ scurvy* because subclinical scurvy can be selective, as it was in the Copenhagen patients.

Scurvy struck selectively in this case also: a surgeon performed exploratory surgery on a 48-year-old California woman in April, 1967 to determine the cause of a painful distended abdomen that had bothered for 5 weeks. She had endured hypermenorrhea for a year but had no unusual bleeding after tooth extractions. She did not bruise easily or exhibit the flat pinhead hemorrhages in the skin or mucous membranes that usually are a first sign of scurvy. The surgeon removed 700 ml [about 3 cups] of loose blood that wasn't confined to arteries and veins. He also removed the appendix, uterus and ovaries.

Being relieved of those body parts failed to provide relief from cramps and indigestion. Four months later, in August, after rapid swelling of the abdomen she was again opened for another look inside. Adhesions that had twisted and constricted the small intestines were cleared away and little spots of blood oozing from tissues were cauterized. About 600 ml of loose blood was removed. She managed to get along without more surgery for 13 months.

Cramps and abdominal distension drove her back to the hospital in September, 1968. She was given packed red cells to normalize the blood picture then opened up again. Three liters of loose blood and clots were removed. Many cyst-like "blisters" on the liver were lanced and drained of blood or clear fluid.

The fix lasted only 2 months. In November the abdominal cavity was not opened, however. Loose blood, almost 2 liters, was removed by suction after insertion of a hollow needle. The same procedure sucked out 2 more liters of blood in January, 1969. Her iron stores were low because of so much blood loss. Her condition baffled the hospital staff. She was given a transfusion and referred to a university medical center.

The staff at the university hospital studied bone marrow and clotting mechanisms thoroughly but saw nothing abnormal. Her abdomen was opened for the fourth time in late January, 1969. About 2.5 liters of loose blood were suctioned away from the various organs. The spleen, being riddled with numerous blood blisters, was considered diseased and removed. Cancer of unknown origin was thought to be the cause of the illness.

The patient returned to the hospital in May, 1969 with the usual complaint of a swollen abdomen, which was opened for the fifth time. A liter of old blood was sucked out. Transfusions were probably given at these last two visits but were not mentioned in the account. They would supply a small amount of vitamin C, along with the hospital diet, so that her response to surgery would appear satisfactory.

And indeed it was, for 13 months. Or perhaps she dreaded another surgery and held out as long as she could. This seems likely because of the volume of blood removed in June, 1970 when her abdomen was opened for the *sixth* time. Nearly 5 quarts of blood that sloshed around outside the vascular system was suctioned out. Tissue supporting the intestines was laced with swollen blood vessels that oozed their contents into the abdominal cavity. No doubt fresh blood was given but this is not mentioned.

She returned to the hospital again in March, 1971 but had no surgery. At that time questions about her diet revealed that she seldom ate fresh fruits and vegetables. Her blood level of C was finally measured. At 0.06 mg/dl, it was well below the level at which signs of scurvy usually appear. A gram of C per day at last brought an end to the surgical excursions that extended over a period of more than 3 years and relieved her of uterus, ovaries, appendix and spleen. [From an item in the *Journal of the American Medical Association*, March 28, 1977, pp1358-9.]

The blood vessels are particularly sensitive to a low C level, as demonstrated by small skin hemorrhages in early scurvy. In this case the bleeding was internal and scurvy is rare enough now to be overlooked while pondering possible causes of a baffling illness. Hippocrates in the fourth century BC advised his students to at least do no harm. The second-century AD version has been attributed to Galen: *"primum non nocere"* [first, do no harm]. Had he known of vitamin C he probably would have added: "second, think of low C, especially if there's bleeding."

We know by now that the requirement for C varies among individuals. On a long sea voyage with little dietary C the high users would die sooner than their shipmates. When Jacques Cartier and 110 men wintered on an island in the St. Lawrence River in 1535-6, 25 had died before the April thaw, 40 more were near death and all but 3 were afflicted with some degree of scurvy.

We assume they left France in good health and all the crew ate the same food. A few either absorbed more of the available C or they used it more efficiently. Fortunately, the captain learned that native people cured scurvy with tea brewed from the bark of a tree thought to have been the white cedar. The remaining men survived. This incident may have been one of the first that led to calling the tree *arbor vitae* [tree of life].

Efficiency of use may be the key to survival. You'll recall the prisoners who used C at different rates, ranging from 2.2% to 4.1% [page 102]. If a person in a group of 9 used almost twice the C as another, how great a difference would be seen in a million? The notion that the RDA suits everyone is fantasy. Even the Russsians didn't care to steal that one. Their daily figure is 125 mg, [15] more than double that clung to by the U.S. for so many years.

In general, women have higher C levels than men and appear to make better use of it in periods of scarcity. During the 9th crusade women were giving birth while men suffered from severe scurvy.[15] A study reported in 1968 found that women, age 20, averaged 1.1 mg of C per deciliter of plasma. The figure for men the same age was 0.8. At age 65 the plasma C in women was 0.75; in men, 0.45,[34] suggesting that the rate of decline with age is equal in both sexes. The low figure for men is in the range where subclinical scurvy may occur. If we project the rate of deline beyond age 65 we see that men will enter true scurvy territory in a few more years.

Some studies don't show as sharp a decline but a measure of white-cell C in another study also found a downward trend in C status with advancing age. 95% of the elderly in institutions were found to have low C, as were 76% of cancer patients and those in hospital, 68% of elderly outpatients and 20% of those who were considered healthy. Only 3% of apparently healthy young individuals had low C levels.[35]

It would seem that a check of C status should be part of routine blood studies upon admission to hospital and its level brought up to the saturation point as a first step on the road to recovery.

People also differ in the amount of oral C that can be tolerated. Cathcart stated that at least 80% of his patients could take 10 to 15 grams a day in divided doses before diarrhea occurred. Of 60 persons studied by another authority, 3 took 20 grams a day without distress. But 2 others experienced intestinal discomfort and diarrhea when only a half gram was taken.[36] Most of the synthetic C on the market is made from corn. Some reactions may be due to an allergy to minute corn residue. Other, more expensive sources of synthetic C are available, such as that made from sugar beets or the starch obtained from sago palm trees.

People differ in the way that C is handled after ingestion, such as the ease of its conversion to oxalate in the gut of those who form stones regularly. Low stomach acidity favors intestinal bacterial species that destroy C. Scurvy has been attributed to such destruction before absorption could occur.[37, 38] Bacterial action may be part of the tolerance effect as well, particularly tolerance that builds up after several months on large doses.

Those who take several grams of C a day without getting diarrhea may notice loose stools after a course of antibiotic therapy. If the looseness persists beyond a week after antibiotics have been discontinued, it may not be due entirely to drugs but to clearance from the gut of bacterial species that had relished C. The amount tolerated before antibiotics is now too much, so that unabsorbed C enters the colon to loosen the stools. The condition is due to osmotic action---attraction and retention of water that otherwise would be absorbed from the colon.

The body can be depleted or deprived of C in many ways. On the subject of deprivation, the multivitamin-mineral tablets that contain both C and copper may conveniently deliver the two nutrients to the stomach but the result is not beneficial. Copper destroys C. They should not be in the same tablet or taken within 2 hours of each other. In his scholarly 3-volume work *Vitamin C* [1989; CRC Press, Boca Raton, FL], C.A.B. Clemetson wrote: "Certainly copper should not be included in vitamin supplements." In *The History of Scurvy & Vitamin C* [1986; Cambridge University Press, Cambridge], K.J. Carpenter wrote that food on British naval ships was cooked in copper kettles but those on merchant ships were iron. The Navy sailors developed scurvy sooner than men on the merchant ships. [Both iron and copper destroy C but copper is far more destructive.]

A diseased intestinal tract deprives by limiting absorption and depletes by being diseased. To list the ways of depletion would be to mention every thing that stresses the body: shock; anxiety; depression; antidepressants; heat; cold; surgery; ulcers; iron overload; smoking; alcohol and substance abuse; poisons; heavy metals; some antibiotics; overexertion; and whatever else is out there.

The depletion that follows a heart attack was studied on 31 patients. The white-cell C level dropped within 12 hours after the event in all 31, enough of a change to cause concern. But the condition wasn't so much a depletion as a relocation of the elite white cells that contained the most C. They all congregated in the heart, so that when blood was drawn for measurement, most of the white cells remaining were the low-C type. Because of the great concentration of white cells, the heart of a patient who dies of the attack contains about a third more C than the heart of someone who dies of a different condition.

In a follow-up study, 6 heart-attack patients received no more C than the diet provided. Plasma and white-cell C dropped far below normal---even to zero in some. The readings were still low 8 weeks later. Each patient in a similar group received a gram of C intravenously every 4 hours for 48 hours, then 2 grams a day orally. Their C levels rose quickly and remained at high normal during the 8-week period. The authors made no comment on how the patients fared [*or did the editor delete it?*] but did state that a low C level is not satisfactory in view of the need for proper tissue repair during recovery.[39, 40] An experiment on dogs revealed that the repair rate of a damaged heart more than doubled when C was administered.[41]

Stroke is another long-term depleter of C. A study reported in 1982 found that stroke victims who died had lower C levels than those who survived. The first one to die had the lowest level. The level remains low for weeks unless supplements are taken.[42]

When a person dies quickly, as in an accident, the body tissues are seen to contain the normal amount of C. When a person dies after long illness the tissues are almost devoid of C.[43]

Among infectious organisms, the champion C depleters may be those that require very high doses to treat. Cathcart reported in 1981 that viral pneumonia, mononucleosis, flu, ECHO virus, candida and bacterial infections require more C than other diseases---up to 200 grams in 24 hours. He wrote of a 98-pound woman who took 2 heaping tablespoons of C every 2 hours for 2 days---a pound, total---to treat mononucleosis. The large amount subdued the virus so that the dose could be lowered to 20 to 30 grams a day for several weeks afterward [ref 5, chapter 1]. His 1984 paper on treating HIV, the AIDS virus, would qualify it to be on the above list also [discussion and reference in chapter 7].

Smoking is a well known depleter of C. A study referenced earlier found that the C levels of smokers were down in the range of persons 40 years older.[34]   Another report informs us that plasma C in smokers is less than half that of nonsmokers.[44] Not all findings are that drastic, however.

Alcohol consumption accounts for low C in two ways: a direct effect on absorption; and low intake due to improper diet by heavy drinkers. Five moderate drinkers whose average daily intake of ethanol was 20 grams or less took a 2-gram dose of C with and without 35 grams of alcohol at breakfast. Alcohol cut the absorption of C almost in half.[45] Regular imbibers might find that keeping the body saturated with C is worthwhile. Ethanol is said to clear out sooner when the C content of the white cells is higher.[46]   And since the nutritional status of the elderly is affected more than that of younger people by moderate drinking,[47] oldsters should take extra C to compensate.

Certain drugs are known depleters of C. Antidepressants and estrogen were mentioned earlier. Diet pills that contained fenfluramine were reported to lower C a generation ago,[48] which probably accounted for reduced demand back then. But a new crop of people with weight problems found the drug effective when manufacturers combined it with phentermine [phen-fen]. Serious side effects resulted in removal of the combination from the market. Whether low C was a factor was not investigated.

Tetracycline lowered both plasma and white-cell C in studies done in 1968 and 1972. Depletion went on for about 36 hours after the drug was discontinued. Three more days passed before the level returned to normal.[49] More C should be taken during such therapy. A second reason for increasing C intake is that the higher intake boosts the effectiveness of certain antibiotics.[50]

Aspirin and C have an interesting relationship. C.W.M. Wilson wrote that taking aspirin increases the uptake of C but drains it from white cells---except when a cold is coming on. At that time, aspirin *enhances* the uptake of C by white cells. After recovery from the cold, aspirin returns to its old habit of draining C from white cells. These studies were done with aspirin doses of from 300 to 900 mg and C doses of from 500 to 2,000 mg.

Aspirin raises plasma C by aiding in its absorption, blocking its uptake by white cells, draining it *from* them, and by blocking some of its excretion by the kidney because aspirin competes with C for use of the same route to leave the body. Even so, higher plasma C translates to increased urinary excretion of it.[48]

Two aspirin taken occasionally won't upset the body's C status but when taken every 6 hours for a week, white-cell C will be lower by 50%. Norman Cousins, the late editor, became ill with a type of arthritis diagnosed as ankylosing spondylitis. His physician said the chance of cure was 1 in 500. Cousins recalled that he was taking 26 aspirin tablets a day plus 4 other drugs.

He was a very sick man. One day, after the outlook seemed hopeless, a dormant instinct must have stirred and thrust up an urge to try a different approach. Or perhaps he remembered reading something about high-dose C therapy. Whatever, he asked to be given 10 grams of C intravenously, plus more the next day and the next, up to 25 grams a day within a week. His physician said that such doses had never been given.

Cousins was the sort of patient we may wish ourselves to be sometimes---bold enough to direct a change in treatment. He could assert himself because he was a Very Important Person. And the doctor was a friend. If his friend had refused Cousins could have announced it to the world with a scathing attack on the doctor-is-God attitude. The old saying that you can never win an argument with a man who has access to ink by the barrel has never been proved scientifically but the doctor didn't wait on science to refute it. He did as directed, not waiting on science to prove the value of C in the case either.

Cousins improved quickly on the regimen, discontinued the pills and soon quit the hospital.[51] In his book about the experience he mentions C only briefly. Most of the credit for his recovery was bestowed on therapeutic laughter and the power of positive thinking.[52]

Such is the lot of vitamin C.

Chapter 6 references

1   Hamil B M, Munks B, Moyer E Z, et al. Vitamin C in the blood and urine of the newborn and in the cord and maternal blood. *Am J Dis Child* 1947; 74:417-33

2   Byerley L O, Kirksey A. Effects of different levels of vitamin C intake on the vitamin C concentration in human milk and the vitamin C intakes of breast-fed infants. *Am J Clin Nutr* 1985; 41:665-71

3   Salmenpera L. Vitamin C nutrition during prolonged lactation: optimal in infants while marginal in some mothers. *Am J Clin Nutr* 1984; 40:1050-56

4   Ingalls T H, Draper R, Teel H M. Vitamin C in human pregnancy and lactation. *Am J Dis Child* 1938; 56:1011-19

5   King C G. Present knowledge of ascorbic acid (vitamin C). *Nutr Rev* 1968; 26:33-6

6   Evans R M, Currie L, Campbell A. The distribution of ascorbic acid between various cellular components of blood in normal individuals, and its relation to the plasma concentration. *Br J Nutr* 1982; 47:473-82

7   Hornig D. Distribution of ascorbic acid, metabolites and analogues in man and animals. *Ann N. Y. Acad Sci* 1975; 258:103-18

8   Szent-Gyorgyi A. Lost in the twentieth century. *Ann Rev Biochem* 1963; 32:1-14

9   Goldsmith G A. Human requirements for vitamin C and its use in clinical medicine. *Ann N.Y. Acad Sci* 1961; 92:230-45

10   Johnson S W, Zilva S S. The urinary excretion of ascorbic and dehydroascorbic acids in man. *Biochem J* 1934; 28:1393-1408

11   Mitra M L. Vitamin-C deficiency in the elderly and its manifestations. *J Am Geriat Soc* 1970; 18:67-71

12   Schorah C J, Newill A, Scott D L, Morgan D B. Clinical effects of vitamin C in elderly patients with low blood-vitamin-C levels. *Lancet* 1979; 1:403-5

13   Andrews J, Letcher M, Brook M. Vitamin C supplementation in the elderly: a 17-month trial in an old persons' home. *Br Med J* 1969; 2:416-8

14   Stevenson N R. Active transport of L-ascorbic acid in the human ileum. *Gastroenterol* 1974; 67:952-6

15   Wilson C W M. Vitamin C. Tissue saturation, metabolism and desaturation. *Practitioner* 1974; 212:481-92

16   Vinson J A, Bose P. Comparative bioavailability to humans of ascorbic acid alone or in a citrus extract. *Am J Clin Nutr* 1988; 48:601-4

17   Yung S, Mayersohn M, Robinson J B. Ascorbic acid absorption in man: influence of divided dose and food. *Life Sciences* 1981; 28:2505-11

18   Zetler G, Seidel G, Siegers C -P, Iven H. Pharmacokinetics of ascorbic acid in man. *Euro J Clin Pathol* 1976; 10:273-82

19   Mickelson O, Keys A. The composition of sweat, with special reference to the vitamins. *J Biol Chem* 1943; 149:479-90

References

20   Kallner A, Hartmann D, Hornig D. Steady-state turnover and body pool of
      ascorbic acid in man. *Am J Clin Nutr* 1979; 32:530-39

21   Kallner A B, Hartmann D, Hornig D. On the requiremants of ascorbic acid
      in man: steady-state turnover and body pool in smokers.
      Am J Clin Nutr 1981; 34:1347-55

22   Hodges R E, Baker E M, Hood J, Sauberlich H E, March S C.
      Experimental scurvy in man. *Am J Clin Nutr* 1969; 22:535-48

23   Hodges R E. What's new about scurvy? *Am J Clin Nutr* 1971; 24:383-4

24   Hodges R E, Hood J, Canham J E, Sauberlich H E, Baker E M.
      Clinical manifestations of ascorbic acid deficiency in man.
      Am J Clin Nutr 1971; 24:432-43

25   Baker E M, Hodges R E, Hood J, et al. Metabolism of 14-C and 3H-labeled
      L-ascorbic acid in human scurvy. *Am J Clin Nutr* 1971; 24:444-54

26   Hornig D, Vuilleumier J -p, Hartmann D. Absorption of large, single, oral
      intakes of ascorbic acid. *Internat J Vit Nutr Res* 1980; 50:309-14

27   Kallner A, Hornig D, Pellikka R. Formation of carbon dioxide from
      ascorbate in man. *Am J Clin Nutr* 1985; 41:609-13

28   Hankes L V, Jansen C R, Schmaeler M. Ascorbic acid catabolism in
      Bantu with hemosiderosis (scurvy). *Biochem Med* 1974; 9:244-55

29   Levine M, Conry-Cantilena C, Wang Y, et al. Vitamin C pharmacokinetics
      in healthy volunteers: evidence for a recommended dietary allowance.
      Proc Natl Acad Sci USA 1996; 93:3704-9

30   Eaton S B, Konner M. Paleolithic nutrition. *N Engl J Med* 1985; 312:283-9

31   Hertog M G L, Kromhout D, Aravanis C, et al. Flavonoid intake and
      long-term risk of coronary heart disease and cancer in the seven countries
      study. *Arch Intern Med* 1995; 155:381-6

32   Jungeblut C. Further observations on vitamin C therapy in experimental
      poliomyelitis. *J Experi Med* 1937; 66:459-77

33   Elmby A, Warburg E. The inadequacy of synthetic ascorbic acid as an
      antiscorbutic agent. *Lancet* 1937; 2:1363-5

34   Brook M, Grimshaw J J. Vitamin C concentration of plasma and
      leukocytes as related to smoking habit, age and sex of humans.
      Am J Clin Nutr 1968; 21:1254-8

35   Basu T K. Schorah C J. *Vitamin C in Health and Disease*
      1982: Croom-Helm Ltd. London

36   Tsao C S. An overview of ascorbic acid chemistry and biochemistry.
      p 35; in *Vitamin C in Health and Disease* Packer L, Fuchs J., editors
      1997; Marcel Dekker, New York

37   Young R M, Rettger L F. Decomposition of vitamin C by bacteria.
      J Bacteriol 1943: 46:351-63

38   Esselen W B Jr., Fuller J E. The oxidation of ascorbic acid as influenced
      by intestinal bacteria. *J Bacteriol* 1939; 37:501-21

Chapter 6 references

39 Hume R, Weyers E, Rowan T, Reid D S, Hillis W S. Leucocyte ascorbic acid levels after acute myocardial infarction. *Br Heart J* 1972; 34:238-43

40 Vallance B D, Hume R, Weyers E. Reassessment of changes in leucocyte and serum ascorbic acid after acute myocardial infarction. *Br Heart J* 1978; 40:64-8

41 Gudbjarnason S, Fenton, J C, Wolf P L, Bing R J. Stimulation of reparative processes following experimental myocardial infarction. *Arch Intern Med* 1966; 118:33-40

42 Hume R, Vallance B D, Muir M M. Ascorbate status and fibrinogen concentrations after cerebrovascular accident. *J Clin Pathol* 1982; 35:195-9

43 Luberoff B J. Symptomectomy with vitamin C. *Chemtech* 1978; Feb:76-86

44 Pelletier O. Smoking and vitamin C levels in humans *Am J Clin Nutr* 1968; 21:1259-67

45 Fazio V, Flint D M, Wahlqvist M L. Acute effects of alcohol on plasma ascorbic acid in healthy subjects. *Am J Clin Nutr* 1981; 34:2394-6

46 Krasner N, Dow J, Moore M R, Goldberg A. Ascorbic-acid saturation and ethanol metabolism. *Lancet* 1974; 2:693-5

47 Jacques P F. Sulsky S, Hartz S C, Russell R M. Moderate alcohol intake and nutritional status in nonalcoholic elderly subjects. *Am J Clin Nutr* 1989; 50:875-83

48 Wilson C W M. Clinical pharmacological aspects of ascorbic acid. *Ann N.Y. Acad Sci* 1975; 258:355-76

49 Windsor A C M, Hobbs S B, Treby D A, Cowper R A. Effect of tetracycline on leucocyte ascorbic acid levels. *Br Med J* 1972; 1:214-5

50 Rawal B D, McKay G, Blackhall M I. Inhibition of Pseudomonas aeruginosa by ascorbic acid acting singly and in combination with antimicrobials: in-vitro and in-vivo studies. *Med J Australia* 1974; 1:169-74

51 Cousins N. Anatomy of an illness (as perceived by the patient) *N Engl J Med* 1976; 295:1458-63

52 Cousins N. *Anatomy of an Illness as Perceived by the Patient: Reflections on Healing and Regeneration.* 1979; Bantam Books, New York.

7

Benefits
Of Extra C

In this chapter the reference accompanies the reported benefit. Other than introducing a little variety, readers are relieved of the task of thumbing and rethumbing pages to learn the source of the information presented. The abbreviated reference notation is sufficient to locate the relevant periodical or book if more information is desired. To most readers of this book for the general public, omitting the names of the authors will not matter, therefore they do not appear, with a few exceptions.

Klenner is one. The North Carolina physician used C as an aid to the treatment of nearly every disease he encountered: all viral diseases; tetanus; severe burns; habitual abortions; barbiturate overdose; snakebite [he preferred it to antivenin]; etc. He gave extra C to pregnant women and their babies. In southeastern U.S., the first quadruple-birth case in which all four survived was under his care. He wrote of a girl, given last rites because of raging mononucleosis, whose recovery was uneventful after her mother, a nurse, added 20 to 30 grams of C to each bottle of intravenous fluid. The attending physician didn't care to use the vitamin in his practice. [*J Appl Nutr* 1971; 23:61-88]

An honors graduate, Klenner, who died in 1984 at age 76, had a master's degree in biology and was a teaching fellow in chemistry while studying for a doctorate in physiology when he switched to medicine. On the first page of the paper referenced above he wrote that during the 1918 flu epidemic the members of his family survived "when scores about us were dying." The Klenners drank a bitter tea brewed from the plant called boneset [*Eupatorium perfoliatum*], a folk medicine for fevers. A good source of C, it gave the family an advantage over the virus.

A Klenner case history from the previous reference: Three boys were accidentally dusted with pesticide from a plane. The older boys covered the youngest so that he did not become ill. The two others were hospitalized. Klenner treated the oldest, age 12, with intravenous C [sodium ascorbate], 10 grams in 50cc of fluid every 8 hours. The boy went home on day 2. The other boy received supportive care only from his physician and died 5 days later.

Another account concerns 3 children with diphtheria who were given different treatments. All received diphtheria antitoxin but only Klenner's patient was given intravenous C, 10 grams diluted 5-to-1 as above, every 8 hours on the first day, every 12 hours on day 2, then a gram orally every 2 hours. His patient lived. The others died.

Next, compare snakebite therapies: A "large highland mocassin" sunk its fangs into the leg of a girl, 7. She was crying and vomiting when seen in emergency 30 minutes later. Klenner injected 4 grams of sodium ascorbate, diluted 5-to-1, his usual preparation. By the time a skin test for antivenin was finished, the child was laughing and drinking orange juice. She was allowed to go home that evening on condition that she be closely monitored during the night. Two more 4-gram injections were given on days 2 and 3, the last at a time when the girl appeared to be completely well. A girl, 16, who was not given C, received 3 doses of antivenin and spent 3 weeks in hospital after being struck in the arm by a mocassin. Her arm swelled to 4 times its normal size. Klenner wrote, "We no longer use anti-venom."

He injected 6 grams of C to start treatment of a girl seriously ill with viral pancreatitis. He would have continued treating but the parents decided to take the child to a university medical center 60 miles distant. Klenner supplied 50 grams of C and phoned ahead to advise how it should be given. When she was seen at the medical center she appeared so well that the physician felt the degree of illness had been overstated. He didn't use the C Klenner had supplied. The child relapsed and spent 2 weeks in hospital. Klenner felt that 2 more injections would have cured the disease.

STROKE

A paper presented at a medical meeting in 1960 mentioned "a late president" who in the final 8 years of his life suffered 6 strokes, the last one fatal. The speaker left it up to the audience to guess which president. He then detailed the results of a study in which bioflavonoids and extra C were used for stroke prevention: 89 patients who'd had 1 or more minor strokes took 600 or 800 mg of C a day along with an equal amount of bioflavonoids to increase uptake and utilization. They were observed for up to 5 years. During the period of observation only 3 minor strokes occurred in the group of 89. Meanwhile, a control group of 62 similar patients who received no extra C or bioflavonoids suffered 30 strokes, 12 minor and 18 severe, of which 5 were fatal [*J Am Geriatric Society* 1961; 9:110].

If those encouraging results had been due to administration of a proprietary substance a dozen scientific trials would have been conducted to determine the optimum dose. Instead, the report has been ignored. Thousands of hapless stroke victims have suffered and died, unaware that supplemental C might have improved their chance for a better life.

A 1995 report pointed to a low C level as a risk factor for stroke [BMJ 6-19-95 p1563] but an accompanying editorial advised reserving judgment until proof by scientific trial. And when will that be? In another 40 years? Medical-journal editors are well aware that trials designed to investigate C objectively are as scarce as their praise of the vitamin.

A 20-year study in Japan also points to low C as a risk factor for stroke. Individuals with the lowest C level due to poor diet had a 70% greater risk of experiencing a stroke than those whose diet included C-rich food, mainly fruits, which kept their C level high [*Stroke* October 2000; 31:2287-94]. On August 2, 2001 the evening medical news informed us that stroke is associated with a high stress level. It shouldn't surprise us. The root of the problem is probably a low C level due to the stress.

DIABETES

The capillaries of diabetics are weaker than normal, a condition exacerbated by low C. Several studies have shown that the capillaries of diabetics can be strengthened with higher C intake. In one such experiment, a group of diabetics took a gram of C a day. A similar group took placebo. Then the groups switched, so that each took extra C for 2 months. The weak capillaries of the members in each group became stronger, almost up to normal, during the time on extra C. Capillary strength deteriorated in 4 of 6 patients after they switched from C to placebo. Small retinal hemorrages occurred in one individual, suggesting that the body had become conditioned to the higher C intake and that a rebound effect occurred when the gram dose was stopped abruptly [*Br Med J* 7-26-75 p 205].

The study was too short to determine whether benefit from C would be permanent. Until patients realize that the dose may need boosting periodically they're at risk of becoming disappointed if the benefit should fade. And never forget individual differences. Some may improve; others may not.

A build-up of sorbitol in red cells causes complications in diabetics. The amount is said to correlate with sorbitol in the eye lens and sciatic nerve, two sites where complications are common. Sorbitol concentration in red cells was seen to be inversely proportional to the amount of C present---the more C, the less sorbitol.

Nondiabetics took 500 mg of C a day for 2 weeks, followed by a 10-day "washout" period in which they took no extra C. Then they took citrus fruit along with 500 mg of C. Significantly more C entered the red cells when taken with citrus. C alone decreased red-cell sorbitol 12.6%. C with citrus decreased it 27.2%, more than twice as much. Sorbitol was reduced 56% in diabetics who took 2 grams of C a day for a time. The same dose taken later by another group of diabetics lowered red-cell sorbitol 44.5 % during a 3-week trial [*Diabetes* 1989; 38: 1036]. Don't get out your stopwatch to determine the time that will pass before diabetics are informed of this. Use geologic time.

Klenner wrote that on 10 grams of C a day, wounds of diabetics heal as well as those of nondiabetics. 60% of his patients on the high dose needed no insulin. The rest managed with less [reference on page 119]. Low C is common in diabetics. They are 2.5 times more stroke-prone than nondiabetics. Taking more C would seem prudent---after first checking for iron overload.

It was mentioned that formula-fed babies are shorted on C from day one [p97]. If susceptible, they're also more prone to develop diabetes on cow-milk formula. This has been suspected for years. A bovine-insulin protein in cow milk can be absorbed into an infant's bloodstream without being split into smaller units. Being foreign, the body's immune system attacks it. The baby's insulin-secreting cells contain a protein that is enough like the foreign protein to prompt the immune system to destroy them also, thereby causing diabetes.

Finnish scientists followed 173 newborns of families whose members were diabetes-prone. About half the babies were given regular cow-milk formula. The other half received formula that had the bovine-insulin protein split into smaller units. By age 2, 10 of the regular-formula babies had developed antibodies to the cow-milk protein, indicating a trend toward diabetes. Only 3 babies who received the split-protein formula developed antibodies.

Another powerful argument against feeding cow-milk to babies comes from a comparison of babies in Cuba and Puerto Rico. Nearly all babies in Cuba are breast-fed. Nearly all babies in Puerto Rico are formula-fed. The number of juvenile-onset diabetes cases in Puerto Rico is **ten times** greater than in Cuba [*Science News*, June 26, 1999]. The additional C in mother's milk is an additional bonus for Cuban babies.

MIGRAINE HEADACHE

The title of a letter to a journal editor is: *Vitamin C and migraine, a case report.* The first sentence reads: "To the Editor: We report here a case in which interrupting an intake of 6 g per day of ascorbic acid resulted in acute onset of headache."

You may now be assuming that another serious side effect of C had been discovered. You would not be alone. The authors of a paper on the safety of antioxidant vitamins also formed that impression [ref 54 chapter 5]. They wrote: "Migraine headaches have been attributed to 6g/d of ascorbic acid in a single case with multiple ascorbic acid challenges."

Let's read the original report to learn just how a person can get a headache by stopping a high dose of C.....We see that migraine headaches had been tormenting a man long before he began to take extra C. *Extra C relieved the headache!* Of course it would return when C was discontinued! To attribute migraine to a lack of controlling medication is ridiculous!

The report concerns a man, 32, who had controlled his headaches for a year with methysergide, sometimes with added codeine, the usual treatment in the 1970s. He tried other methods of obtaining relief, among them extra C. Within two months he was taking 6 grams of C a day and had discontinued other drugs. Headaches occurred only when he failed to take the morning dose of C.

His skeptical physician arranged a double-blind test in order to rule out the placebo effect. The man was given 8 packets of pills, each containing 6 grams of C; and 7 packets containing dummy pills. He was to choose any packet for the day's medication, record the time of day taken and severity of head-ache, if any. He was allowed to take his own C on any day the medication was ineffective. On 3 days he did so. When the code was broken at the end of the test it was seen that he had correctly identified all the days he had taken dummy pills, including those when severe headaches drove him to take his own C [*N Engl J Med* 1978; 299:364].

The authors of the above letter speculated that the spell of headaches was about to end when treatment with extra C began, therefore its intake could not be reduced without causing head-aches. A reluctance to attribute benefit to C is the mother of hypothetical excess. This wild guess occurred during the 1970s when every critic of extra C was trying to shoot it down.

The amount of C used in the above case failed to relieve a friend's headache. He didn't consider increasing the dose.

MULTIPLE SCLEROSIS

Circumstantial evidence suggests that an infectious agent, probably viral, initiates multiple sclerosis in susceptible people. Leather tanners and meat handlers have more than their share of the disease. Scientists who examined the brains of sick sheep contracted it. Meat brought to the Faroe Islands was blamed for cases that occurred there. Patients have high antibodies to cer-tain viruses [S. D. Cook, *Handbook of Multiple Sclerosis*; Marcel Dekker, New York, 1990]. One virus is almost always present [*Proc Natl Acad Sci USA* 1997; 94:7583]. It may be the one that causes flare-ups, as all patients experiencing them had viral par-ticles in plasma at the times [*Lancet* 1998; 352:1033].

In 1947, 9 MS patients who improved on a C-rich diet had low levels beforehand---lower than all except 2 of 11 hospi-talized patients [*Med Times* 1947; 75:189; and *Med Record* 1947; 160:661]. Another MS group also perked up on extra C [*Geriatrics* 1954; 9:375]. In 1982 MS patients were said to have chronic subclinical scurvy. A trial to demonstrate the value of extra C was urged [*Med Hypoth* 1982; 9:635].   ......Fat chance.

Recently Borna disease virus [more about it later] was seen to be active in 2 of 19 MS patients during flare-ups. Antibodies to it were found in 13% of MS patients [*Lancet* 1998; 352:1828]. Some patients say they are helped by bee stings. The therapy may work by stimulating the immune system, although MS is considered to be an autoimmune disease in which the immune system attacks body tissue, the nerve sheath in this disease. John

K. Wolf, in *Mastering Multiple Sclerosis*, 2nd edition [1987; Academy Books, Rutland, VT] advises that 4 to 8 grams of C a day be taken to acidify the urine.

Advances in technology soon may find the reason some scientists who examined the brains of sick sheep developed MS. The connection may have been merely coincidence because the spongy-brained sheep had scrapie, which has a stronger connection with "mad-cow disease" and Cruetzfeldt-Jakob disease, a similar condition in humans. A spongy brain is common to those 3 diseases but not MS. The new variant of the human disease appears to have been the result of an infectious agent, a rogue prion, harbored by sheep with scrapie whose byproducts were fed to cattle whose beef was eaten by humans.

There's a report that a tiny virus-like particle linked to scrapie has been detected; and a later report that identical particles were detected in Creutzfeldt-Jakob brains [*Lancet* 1994; 343:894 & 344:923]. Some scientists feel that the rogue prion protein was turned from its path of righteousness by a virus lurking somewhere [*Lancet* 2000; 355:192]. It was mentioned in chapter 3 that viral components were found in *healthy* bone-marrow cells of multiple-myeloma patients, not affected ones. Remote control by a virus may exist in other diseases also. And massive doses of C could be of value, as it was in the case of multiple myeloma.

PARKINSON'S DISEASE
A 62-year-old man with Parkinson's disease improved after being started on levodopa but later was unable to take enough of it because of nausea. He stopped the 4-gram dose, then started again with 3 grams a day. The amount was barely effective. He was started on a gram of C a day which was increased gradually to 4 grams while the daily dose of levodopa was cut to 2 grams. Within a month the man could move his head better and play the organ again, an ability he had lost several years before. A double-blind test was arranged to determine whether the benefit was due to placebo effect. The man reverted to his previous con-

dition. He improved again after resumption of C. The authors wrote that further study is warranted [*Lancet* 1975; 1:527].

Around 1920 a viral encephalitis caused aftereffects that mimicked Parkinson's so closely the two could not be separated by examination of brain tissue. True Parkinson's doesn't appear to be associated with a virus---but the limits of the operating mode of viruses has not yet been determined.

In the fall of 1989 selegeline, trademarked Deprenyl in the U.S., received extensive press coverage as a welcome edition to treatments for Parkinson's. An article stated that further research will include its use in combination with vitamin E. One might wonder why E was chosen when there's a published account of benefit from C and a published account of no benefit from E.

The failure of E involves a horse trainer who took 400 units a day because the vitamin seemed to improve the speed of horses. The first signs of Parkinson's appeared at age 56. At 58 he began to take levodopa. Taking E for 20 years failed to prevent the disease or alter its course afterward [*Lancet* 2-28-87 p 508].

Another trial with E, 2,000 to 3,000 units, did include 3 grams of C daily, with encouraging results. The combination delayed the need for levodopa or Deprenyl 2.5 years, on average. A man in the group managed to avoid drugs for 8 years [*Ann Neurol* 1992; 32s:128]. It is doubtful that a study with bowel-tolerance intake of C will ever be conducted but it should be.

CATARACTS

The lenses of a man in his middle 30s were clouding so that his vision decreased to 20/40. A medical check-up found no abnormalities. He was started on 4 grams of C a day. Four months later his lenses were clear; visual acuity 20/20. He was then advised to discontinue the dose but declined. When last seen 13 years later he was still taking the 4-gram dose and had no problems [*N Engl J Med* 1972; 287:412].

High-dose C probably would not reverse clouded lenses in older persons. An elderly woman I know developed them while taking 7 grams of C a day. But she had been taking hydrocortisone for years, a drug conducive to cataract formation. Her dose of C may have been somewhat protective, however, as she reached 84 before needing lens replacement in one eye.

Cataracts occur in lenses that have a low level of C [*Int J Vit Nutr Res* 1986; 56:165]. The report was not fresh news; a 1954 report linked low C and cataracts [*Arch Ophthalmol* 1954; 51:1]. They appear to develop as the C content of the lens declines [*Ann N.Y. Acad Sci* 1987; 498:307]. People who do not take vitamins, including 300 to 600 mg of C a day, are 4 times more likely to develop cataracts [*Ann N.Y. Acad Sci* 1989; 570:372].

The results of studies on cataracts are reaching people who can benefit, as the May/June 1999 issue of *Modern Maturity* reported the risk of developing them was 80% lower in women who had taken 400 mg or more of C a day for 10 or more years. It has been suggested that cortical cataracts, the type that forms in the soft outer part of the lens, may be due to slow movement of C into eye fluid [*Ophthalmic Res* 1988; 20:164]. Whether a higher blood level of C would prevent them is not known.

The eyes of animals active in daylight contain more C than eyes of nocturnal animals. Daylight is said to be more stressful to eyes and the higher concentration of C provides protection and speeds repair of damage [*Arch Ophthalmol* 1986; 104:753].

SUGAR AND THE ELDERLY

Older persons don't handle sugar as well as when they were younger. The inability is somewhat related to the blood level of C, as seen in the following report: Oldsters were divided into 2 groups, those with a C level of 0.6 or more and those having a lower level. After an overnight fast, individuals in the higher C group had a blood glucose level that was nearer normal. Both groups then took a glucose-tolerance test. The higher-C group controlled their sugar better, having 10% to 14% lower glucose levels than were seen in the low-C group [*J Am Geriatric Soc* 1965; 13:924].

VIRAL HEPATITIS

Several reports mentioned in chapter 1 involved successful use of C for viral hepatitis. Klenner called C the drug of choice for the disease. His massive oral and IV doses were given simultaneously. The IV amount ranged from 400 to 600 mg per kilogram of body weight every 8 to 12 hours along with 10 grams a day orally in divided doses. At 600 milligrams per kilogram a 155-pound patient would receive 42 grams every 8 hours---126 grams a day. Dosing did not extend beyond a week because patients were well by then [*J Applied Nutr* 1971; 23:61-88].

The highest dose Klenner reported using was not for hepatitis but as 2 injections of 1,200 mg per kilogram of body weight for puerperal sepsis before reducing to half that amount. The day may come when infectious agents will have acquired resistance to all antibiotics. Massive amounts of intravenous C may be necessary then. Already hepatitis-B virus mutants are turning up in vaccinated individuals [*Lancet* 2000; 355:812].

Edward Greer, a physician who treated with high doses, used a commercial product that contained large amounts of C to counter viral hepatitis in a young woman. His comment: "...the most dramatic recovery from hepatitis that I have ever observed." [*J Indiana Med Assoc* 1962; 55:1151.]

Cathcart wrote that chronic hepatitis in which the virus is well entrenched in liver cells cannot actually be cured with high-dose C but can be controlled. Whether infusion of massive doses day and night for several weeks would result in a cure will not be known until someone tries the regimen.

HIGH CHOLESTEROL AND/OR HEART DISEASE

Epidemiological studies---observations of population groups in order to determine factors that cause, or help resist, disease, are a useful beginning in the effort to better our health. From them we learn of the "Mediterranean diet" in which olive oil helps protect the vascular system; and the "French paradox" in which a high-fat diet is neutralized somewhat by the antioxidants and alcohol in red wine.

Learning how a substance works is the next step. How does a diet rich in C promote cardiovascular health? Long before antioxidant became a household word, scientists saw that 50 in a group of 60 people with heart or vascular problems who took 1.5 to 3 grams of C a day for up to 30 months exhibited improvement that ranged from moderate to impressive [*J Am Geriatric Soc* 1996; 14:1239]. More recently it was seen that an orange a day, about 80 mg of C plus flavonoids, lowered the risk of heart attack by 10% [*BMJ* 6-19-95 p 1559]. ...How?

Healthy volunteers took 2 grams of C. Its plasma level peaked 2 hours afterward at 2 mg/dl, up from 0.8 at the start. [A 4-gram dose boosted the level to an unexpected 3.5 mg/dl but was not used in the study.] After observing the effect of the 2-gram dose in healthy persons, it was given to patients with coronary artery disease. A similar group took placebo.

Two hours after ingestion the main artery of an arm was examined by ultrasound to determine whether any change had occurred. The arteries of the C group had dilated significantly more than those in the placebo group. The investigators concluded that C causes blood vessels to dilate, thus allowing greater blood flow [*Circulation* 1996; 93:1107]. ...How?

It has something to do with the effect of C on cells that line blood vessels, causing them to release nitric oxide, Nature's own nitroglycerin fix. However, the *antioxidant* effect of C, not nitric oxide, was said to account for the restoration of normal blood flow in smokers' hearts when 3 grams of C were taken [*Lancet* 2000; 356:1007]. Preventing blood components from clumping may be another way that C lowers the risk of having a heart attack. Less clumping occurs when a gram of C is taken after a high-fat meal. People with hyperlipidemia, a high-blood-fat condition, exhibited less blood clumping while taking 3 grams of C a day [*Clin Cardiol* 1985; 8:552].

The how of it needn't concern people with cardiovascular problems, though. All they need to know is that C is beneficial.

BLOOD VESSEL FLEXIBILITY

A normal blood vessel expands about 15% when the heart beats, then contracts until the next beat repeats the cycle. Expansion is reduced when hardening of the arteries occurs, thereby putting more load on the heart. After learning that 2 grams of C restored a bit of flexibility to diseased blood vessels [preceding page], researchers gave 500 mg of C a day for a month to heart patients whose vessel expansion had averaged 6.6%. The dose increased vessel expansion to 9%, on average. No increase was seen in the placebo group [*Science News* 1999; 156:21].

PAGET'S DISEASE OF BONE

Also called *osteitis deformans*, a disease of middle age and up. Around our bones we have bone-building cells and bone-removal cells. Normally they are supervised by a biological foreman of some sort so that all goes well. In this disease the building and dismantling occur at random, causing thickened, bowed or weakened bones, sometimes along with a considerable amount of pain.

Detection techniques indicate that foreign matter in the unsupervised cells belongs to a virus. When a virus or a pain is involved, think of vitamin C. A research group did. They gave 16 patients 3 grams of C a day for 2 weeks to check on its ability to control pain. Three patients, including one who had endured pain for 15 years, experienced complete relief. Pain eased off a bit in 5 others but the remaining 8 were not helped [*Acta Vitamin Enzymol* (Milano) 1978; 32:45]. Larger doses were not tried. We long for the day when using bowel-tolerance doses becomes standard procedure.

HEALTHIER GUMS

At the 1998 meeting of the International Association for Dental Research, low-C diets were said to increase the risk of periodontal disease, moreso in smokers. Advised daily intakes: a gram of calcium and 2 grams of C [*Let's Live* Jan. 1999].

ENHANCED FERTILITY

Couples ought to try extra C first rather than hormones that may result in a litter. The inability to conceive is sometimes due to the clumping of sperm so that they don't get on with the job of finding the egg. The humorous answer to the question of why so many sperm are needed [they don't ask directions either] may have a more appropriate explanation: they like to hang out together, a male-bonding tendency. Extra C breaks up the party.

A group of men unable to get their wives pregnant had an average serum C level of 0.2 mg/dl, a figure down in the pre-scurvy range. Their semen C level was also low, averaging 4.2 mg/dl. On average, 37% of their sperm clumped. A week on 500 mg of C every 12 hours [a gram a day], raised the serum C level to 1.3 mg/dl. Semen C rose to 12.7 mg/dl. Sperm clumping declined to 14%. After 3 weeks on the regimen clumping had declined to 11%.

A man is considered infertile when clumping is greater than 20%. The researchers calculated that at the rate the men improved, the gram of C a day would have restored fertility in 4 days. They found a direct link between serum and semen C levels. Infertility would occur if serum C should drop to around 0.4 mg/dl. Clumping would practically disappear over time if serum C level were maintained at 0.9 mg/dl [*Journal of the American Medical Association* 1983; 249:2747].

STUBBORN BLADDER INFECTION

An abnormal urinary bladder lining, termed malacoplakia, was seen in a woman with recurring bladder infection. The condition was thought to be permanent. After 6 years of intermittent antibiotic therapy, 500 mg of C taken 4 times a day were added to the regimen. The disturbing symptoms vanished within 6 weeks. The woman reduced her C intake to a gram a day 6 months later. An examination at month 9 found the bladder lining to be normal. It was still normal at month 18 [*J Urol* 1983; 130:1174].

MENTAL ILLNESS

Borna disease virus usually targets animals, causing them to behave oddly. Horses, cattle, sheep and cats have persistent infections. Susceptible humans can be infected also. More than half of a group of schizophrenics had traces of the virus [*Lancet* 1997; 349:1813]. It has also been recovered from patients with depression, obsessive-compulsive disorder and chronic fatigue syndrome. Virus taken from humans has caused Borna disease in animals [*Molecular Psychiatry* 1996; 1:200].

Nucleic acid fractions of the virus were found in the blood of a man with paranoia and other delusions who'd complained of aches, dizziness and sleep disorder for 28 years. It suggests that humans, like animals, are also subject to persistent infections, which can flare up to cause acute illness [*Lancet* 1998; 352:623].

One would expect that an antiviral drug could treat mental illness caused by a virus. It has. A depressed patient known to be infected with Borna disease virus began to improve during the second week of treatment with the antiviral drug amantadine and was entirely free of symptoms by day 15 [*Lancet* 1997; 349:178]. One would expect C to do as well. In the days before a viral connection was suspected, a gram of C an hour restored a schizophrenic to normal in 2 days [*Dis Nerv Sys* 1963; 24:273].

Components from viruses other than that which causes Borna disease have been detected in the human nervous system. Of first-episode schizophrenia cases in young adults, 30% exhibited a rise in retrovirus activity. The virus may have been lurking in the human genome for eons [*Science News* 2001; 159:228; and *Discover*, October 2001 pp 33-34].

Viral activity may explain why schizophrenics needed to take an average of 40 grams of C a day to produce a color change in a urine test while nonschizophrenics changed the color on only 4 grams a day [*Int J Neuropsychiat* 1966; 2:204]. More cases of schizophrenia occur in areas of low-C intake [*Human Nutr Clin Nutr* 1986; 40C:421]. Ten of 13 schizophrenics improved on 8 grams of C a day [*J Clin Psychopharmachol* 1987; 7:282].

TOXINS AND POISONOUS BITES

As mentioned, Klenner used extra C to counter snakebite venom and pesticide poisoning. Black-widow spider bites were treated also. A girl, not yet 4, was seen the morning after a bite on the abdomen the previous evening. She had vomited, was stuporous, with labored breathing and temperature of 103.4. Klenner gave calcium gluconate first, then 4 grams of C 15 minutes later, both intravenously. At hour 6 the fever was 101. Several more shots plus oral C over the next 3 days brought the child back to normal. The bite on so small a child was considered life threatening [*Tristate Med J* 12-15-57 p 15].

Edward J Calabrese reviewed the early and recent literature [to 1980] on the use of C to reduce toxic symptoms due to pesticides, herbicides, heavy metals, hydrocarbons, radiation, gases, common drugs, heat and cold [*Nutrition and Environmental Health, volume 1---the Vitamins* John Wiley & Sons; New York; 1980]. He mentioned the depletion of C by bacterial toxins; the protection of lab animals from irritating chemicals by C; that clearance of chlorinated hydrocarbons is slower in C-deficient rats; and that extra C counters the effects of malathion and parathion in rats. Extra C was protective against all the toxins noted.

In the days when syphilis was treated with an arsenic compound, extra C was shown to decrease the side effects without interfering with the curative power. C countered the toxicity of cadmium, cobalt, vanadium, copper, selenium, and fluoride but was said to increase toxicity of cyanide. The pitting and mottling of teeth by drinking water that contained excessive amounts of fluoride was worse in children having lower C levels.

In some studies, extra C protected against toxicity from lead, an occupational disease in early painters, but others found no benefit from the small amount of C tested. A later study found it to be effective in removing lead from the nervous system of rats. [Keeping the C level high might protect children against excess lead in the environment today.]

Mercury reduces tissue levels of C. C-making animals make less C in the presence of mercury. An injection of mercury cyanide that killed all guinea pigs in a group could kill only 60% of those given the human equivalent of 35 grams of C. The risk of cardiac death was said to be diminished when extra C was taken along with diuretics that contained mercury.

A number of studies have shown that extra C reduces the effect of exposure to benzene, which causes bleeding signs similar to scurvy. Toxicity of other hydrocarbons is also reduced by C. PCB toxicity in guinea pigs is "markedly alleviated" when extra C is given. Extra C protects people who work with TNT and vinyl chloride.

That C reduces the formation of nitrosamines was mentioned earlier. Another nitrate problem involves susceptible infants who are at risk of having nitrate converted to nitrite in the gut. The nitrite than combines with hemoglobin to produce methemo-globin, which doesn't carry oxygen. Extra C has been used to treat the condition. A mouse study indicates that C can treat ozone toxicity.

C has antihistaminic properties. Exposure to various dusts raises the blood level of histamine which reduces the ability to breathe easily. Workers who took 500 mg of C a day for a week exhibited only half the distress of a control group, as measured by forced expiratory volume per second. And in a noisy workplace, people who took 100 mg of C after lunch outper-formed a control group in coordination, reaction speed and endurance. As should be expected, their superiority did not carry over to the following day.

In addition to the Calabrese review, three Australians, Glen Dettman, PhD, Ian Dettman, PhD and Archie Kalokerinos, MD, have collected items on C versus toxins and poisons. Their com-bined investigative and clinical experience resulted in the book *Vitamin C   Nature's Miraculous Healing Missile!* [Frederick Todd; Melbourne; 1983]. They wrote of 3 men who were given

2 grams of C intravenously for snakebite as emergency treatment in a Colombia oil company hospital in 1947. Symptoms diminished immediately. Repeat injections were given every 3 hours until no longer needed.

Another report involves tetanus toxin given to dogs. It saddens me to contemplate the results of these experiments on dogs, even though they were done years ago. But as long as they were done, spreading the knowledge gained honors them more than ignoring it. All dogs given a certain amount of toxin died in 47 to 65 hours. All dogs in a second group survived with only mild symptoms when given the toxin along with a gram of C per kilogram of body weight twice a day for 3 days. A third group had no reaction at all when C was given for 3 days prior to, and 3 days after, the dose of toxin. Administration of C was delayed in another group for 40 to 47 hours after the dogs had received toxin. They survived but exhibited "marked symptoms of the disease."

Several years ago a physician friend successfully treated a human case of tetanus with heroic supportive measures around the clock for more than a week. Extra C was not part of the treatment because the medical community was not aware of the antitoxic nature of C. The high cost of the treatment was not questioned by the insurance company that paid the bill. It might have been, had the officials known that a gram of C per kilogram of body weight infused twice a day along with a little calcium would have cured the patient in less than half the time.

SCORPION STING: FIVE-HOUR DRAMA

An account in *Reader's Digest*, October 1995, concerns a family vacationing in Mexico when their toddler son was stung by a scorpion. The nearest antivenin was in Tucson, about 185 miles north in Arizona. During the next 5 hours while the boy's condition deteriorated he was rushed by car, ambulance and helicopter to the hospital. We assume the parents were deeply grateful for the injection of antivenin, which may have saved the

boy's life.   Their emotions would not have been so positive if
the child had died enroute and they'd have learned that a gram of
C in a single injection gave prompt relief from a scorpion sting!
[*Arch Pediat* 1952; 69:151.]   Two or three grams orally would
do as well.

The above information should have been common knowledge
for 50 years! Instead, the bias against C that sustains an ongoing
disregard for its life-saving potential has probably been
responsible for hundreds of preventable fatalities.

An unhappy cobra's bite provided the drama for the *Digest*
two months later. In spite of many doses of antivenin the man
hovered near death for days. There would have been no drama if
those involved in treatment had known of the excellent record of
C against toxins. A "killer-bee" multiple-sting case made TV
news in late summer, 2001. Someday, I'm sure, someone will
ease the misery of that trauma with high-dose C.

One wonders whether C could neutralize the so-called nerve
gases that may be used in war or by vindictive groups. We doubt
the World Trade Center disaster will prompt a study of C for the
purpose but it should. Bowel-tolerance doses should be tried
against anthrax toxin also. We are in great danger of smallpox
virus as a weapon, an expert said, because of low vaccine supplies and no treatment for the disease. I believe the millions of
people who have extra C on hand---and who know how to take it
properly---are well prepared for any viral or toxin-producing
bacterial attack. The available vaccines and antiviral drugs
could be saved for the 20% who are not able to take therapeutic
doses of C. Stockpiling injectable C would help also.

ASTHMA

Oxidant stress is high in the lungs of asthmatics, indicating a
need for a plentiful source of antioxidants. The lung surfaces of
mild asthmatics have low levels of vitamins C and E. Their
plasma and white cells have low C levels. Increasing C intake
reduces the severity of attacks [*Lancet* 1999; 354:482].

POST-FRACTURE DISCOMFORT

A complication of broken bones termed *post-traumatic dystrophy* afflicts a percentage of people who are on the mend from fractures. Netherland scientists wrote: "There are very few substances that have such an impact on wounds after burns and the signs of inflammation at that stage as vitamin C." Aware of this, they gave 500 mg of C a day for 50 days to patients with wrist fractures to see if C would have the same impact on post-traumatic dystrophy. It did, even at the relatively low dose. The condition occurred in 22% of those who took placebo but in only 7% of those on C [*Lancet* 1999; 354:2025].

GALLBLADDER DISEASE

The observation that guinea pigs with low C levels tend to develop gallstones led to the thought that low C might be a factor in the human condition also. An epidemiological survey of 13,130 U.S. adults found that more gallbladder disease was indeed associated with a low C level---but only in women. Women who took C supplements had less gallbladder trouble. Men were not significantly affected [*Arch Intern Med* 2000; 160:931].

DEEP VEIN THROMBOSIS

One of the hazards older hospitalized patients face is the possibility of a clot in a leg vein due to inactivity while lying in bed. Preventives such as anticoagulants, elastic stockings and intermittent-pressure devices are used. Extra C is of value also. A double-blind study found that clots occurred in 60% of patients given the usual care while only 33% of those taking a gram of C a day developed them *Lancet* 1973; 2:199]. In view of the fact that most of an oral dose of C has left the bloodstream 6 hours after ingestion, the gram performed impressively during its short stay. It would be interesting to see the results of a study in which a gram would be given every 3 hours. Frequent dosing would also increase the low C level that is seen in most hospitalized patients. The higher level should speed recovery.

CRIB DEATH

Dr. Kalokerinos' book *Every Second Child* [Thomas Nelson, Melbourne, 1974; and Keats, New Canaan, CT, 1981] is distributed in the U.S. by a group trying to get the word out that cases of sudden infant death syndrome [SIDS] can be reduced dramatically, as Kalokerinos had shown, simply by giving babies a small amount of C. He had noticed that illness usually precedes SIDS. Babies haven't much reserve capacity for C so that illness drains their little bodies quickly. Whether low C has anything to do with an abnormal electrocardiogram that is said to be associated with half of SIDS cases [*Lancet* 2001; 357:889] or a diminished reflex to breathe is not known but it *is* known that illness lowers the C level, which can lead to more problems.

HYPERTENSION

In a randomized trial a placebo was ineffective while 500 mg of C a day for a month lowered the mean blood pressure of hypertensive patients 9%. Persons with normal blood pressure were not affected [*Lancet* 1999; 354:2048]. The reduction may be due to artery dilation mentioned on page 130. The study was not long enough to determine whether the tolerance effect would kick in and require a rise in dose to maintain benefit.

EYE IRRITATION

Antihistamines and other medication failed to relieve the sore eyes of an associate professor of biology who felt that extra C is unnecessary. But she decided to try it. Relief occurred within a week after she began taking 500 mg a day [*Am J Pub Hlth* 1982; 72:1412]. Extra C *is* necessary for some individuals.

PRE-ECLAMPSIA

141 women were given a gram of C and 400 units of E a day after it was determined that they were at risk of developing pre-eclampsia. Of those on C/E, 8% developed the condition, vs 17% of 142 women on placebo [*Lancet* 1999; 354:810].

CHROMATE DERMATITIS
Barrier creams were useless and gloves a handicap to a radiologist who was sensitive to chromate in developing solutions. Dramatic improvement occurred in 3 weeks when he applied 10% C in petroleum jelly to his hands 3 times a day. The dermatitis vanished in 2 months. After 15 months he was able to discontinue treatment [*Contact Derm* 1984; 10:252].

STRONGER IMMUNITY
More rapid movement of white cells to areas in the body where they were needed occurred when 2 grams of C a day were taken. A rise to 3 grams daily caused an even greater response [*Am J Clin Nutr* 1980; 33:71.   Two months of antibiotic treatment failed to cure a diabetic's ear infection. His white cells were sluggish.   When given 3 grams of C a day the man's infection cleared up in 7 weeks [*Arch Otolaryngol* 1982; 108:122].   Other reports on the use of extra C to boost the immune reaponse are in the literature.   C may also work indirectly by reducing the viral count in the body.   Viruses are said to tie up the body's supply of selenium, another booster of the immune response [*Lancet* 2000; 356:235].   A reduced number of viruses would allow greater selenium activity.

LONGER LIFE
An epidemiological study in California revealed that men who took from 300 to 600 mg of C a day lived an average 6 years longer than men who took no more than 50 mg a day. The average for women on the higher doses was a year longer.   An increased intake of C was more conducive to a longer life than lower cholesterol or lower fat intake [*Epidemiol* 1992; 3;194].

ARTHRITIC KNEES
Low C is a risk factor [*Lancet* Sept 8, 01 p775]. Worsening is retarded by taking 3 or more times the RDA of C [*Arth & Rheu* 1996; 39:648]. Other joints probably would benefit also.

BETTER HEALTH

Dr. Emanuel Cheraskin, a physician and dentist has written extensively on C.   In *Vitamin C: Who Needs It?* [Arlington Press, Birmingham, AL; 1993], he wrote that in the 1970s his group questioned 1083 dentists and their spouses about their diet and vitamin intake.   They were then asked to answer 195 questions about their health.   After the data was processed it was seen that as the mean amount of C ingested rose toward 410 mg a day, the amount of poor-health signs and symptoms declined.

MEGALOBLASTIC ANEMIA IN PREGNANCY

Textbooks list many causes of megaloblastic anemia.   Among them are malabsorption; lack of vitamin B12; lack of intrinsic factor [see chapter 5]; lack of folic acid; and having a fish tapeworm that consumes B12.   The disease is treated with B12, intrinsic factor and folinic acid, a form of folic acid the body can use.

Vitamin C is said to aid in the conversion of folic acid to folinic acid.   Clemetson wrote that physicians have cured cases of megaloblastic anemia that accompanied scurvy simply by administering C [*Vitamin C, Vol II*; CRC Press, Boca Raton, FL; 1989].   In 3 cases of megaloblastic anemia during pregnancy, neither B12 nor C given separately was effective but were curative when given together.   Another case was cured with folic acid when B12 alone was not effective [*Proc Soc Experi Biol Med* 1951; 78:238].   In that case, enough C must have been available to help convert folic acid to folinic acid.

C GETS THE LEAD OUT;   REDUCES TOOTH DECAY

An item in *Science News*, 6-26-99, condenses some reports indicating that more C and calcium in children's diet would lower the accumulation of lead.   Lead, which has been linked to anemia and mental retardation, also stunts the growth of salivary glands.   This results in a drier mouth that favors tooth decay.   C and calcium tie up the lead so that it is eliminated, not absorbed.

ALZHEIMER'S DISEASE

Amyloid, a "sludge protein" accumulates in the brains of pateints with Alzheimer's disease, interfering with function. A study with mice to determine whether C could clear away the amyloid reported no benefit. But a second study found that C was indeed capable of eliminating the substance [*Br J Experi Pathol* 1985; 66:137]. Amyloid mice given C far outlived a control group [*Arth & Rheu* 1987; 30:718].

It is not known whether any findings with mice would apply to humans but there's good reason to take extra C because patients with senile dementia have low blood levels of C and folic acid [*Br Med J* 1985; 1:1234]. Many oldsters harbor cold-sore virus in the areas of the brain that are affected by Alzheimer's. It has been suggested that brain damage occurs whenever the virus becomes active---a chipping away of the senses. Starting treatment early, as advocated by an authority [*Time*, July 17, 2000] might be a good idea. Persons having the ε4 variant of the apoe gene are said to be more apt to develop Alzheimer's [some say earlier] and the risk is even greater if the cold-sore virus is present in the brain [*Molec/Chem Neuropath* 1996; 39:648]. Worse, persons who are susceptible to cold sores are more apt to have the variant gene. This synergy effect has been questioned, however [*Lancet* 7-18-98 p238 and 10-17-98 p1312]. More and more is being reported about risk factors in our genetic make-up. When the ε4 variant is linked to a particular area on chromosome 10, the risk of getting the disease is 16 times greater [*Molec Psychiat* 2001; 6:413].

HEROIN DETOXIFICATION

Cathcart mentioned a Los Angeles physician who detoxified heroin addicts quickly with 60 grams of C a day. They experienced no withdrawal symptoms. Heroin taken during treatment had no effect [*Chemtech* 1978; Feb. p 76]. If the remedy is that simple why hasn't it spread as quickly as the addiction? One might suspect that money is somehow involved.

EHLERS-DANLOS SYNDROME

This is a rare hereditary condition with several types of collagen abnormalities. Bones can be fragile and skin as stretchy as rubber. In some types, tissues bruise easily. C is required for the formation of good collagen, therefore it was thought that extra C might be of value in this disease. Four grams were given for 2 years to a boy, 8, with a type 6 abnormality. Lung capacity and wound healing improved but the skin remained fragile and the bones continued to be flexible. Higher doses were not tried [*J Pediat* 1978; 92:378].

CHEDIAK-HIGASHI SYNDROME

This is another rare hereditary condition. White-cell chemistry and function are abnormal, allowing frequent infections. No effective treatment exists. The condition improved in a year-old baby who was given 200 mg of C for 2 months [*N Engl J Med* 1976; 295:1041].

Meniere's syndrome was relieved by extra C [*J Laryngol & Otol* 1939; 54:256].

Nerve deafness slowly improved on vitamins B, C and bioflavonoids [*Mayo Clinic Proc* 1962; 37:474].

Rheumatic fever joint pain and fever either vanished or diminished in 7 cases on 4 grams of C a day [*N Engl J Med* 1950; 242:614].

Brucellosis, also called Mediterranean, Malta, undulant or intermittent fever, responds to C if the victim hasn't been helped by vaccination. Twelve cases on 3 or 4 grams a day improved markedly [*Arch Pediat* 1955; 72:119].

Various conditions in which extra C yielded "spectacular results" are noted, among them scarlet fever, tuberculosis and pelvic inflammation. "...toxins are rapidly neutralized and the febrile process...is abated, usually within a few hours..." [*Arch Pediat* 1952; 69:151]. The resurgence of tuberculosis worldwide should prompt an objective clinical study with C.

POLIOMYELITIS

Vaccines have nearly eliminated polio but the history of treating it with C is enlightening. The knowledge could come in handy someday. In the last half of the 1930s, studies with monkeys suggested that C might prevent crippling. Although some studies yielded inconclusive results, others showed that C could prevent crippling and death in a good percentage of the animals. But in 1939 a virologist reported that C was of no value at all against the virus. His verdict dried up funding for further experiments.

Klenner wrote in 1952 that the final experiment used more virus and less C, a "blunder" [?] to which "Thousands of children owe their paralyzed limbs..."

While they waited for something patentable.

Klenner had the experience to support his criticism. In 1948 he brought 60 children through a polio epidemic without a death or crippling. His intramuscular shots of C ranged as high as 2 grams every 2 hours around the clock, age and fever determining the dose. A girl in his neighborhood whose doctor did not use C ended up in braces.

Intramuscular shots of C are painful. Klenner applied ice to the buttocks before and after to ease the sting. Another physician, Edward Greer, treated polio with oral doses. His own daughter responded so well that C was discontinued after only a day---but had to be resumed when fever returned. Some of Greer's patients did not respond as quickly. He treated one case with 10 grams of C every 3 hours for 10 days before the virus was subdued. The 3-hour schedule tells us that Dr. Greer was familiar with the nature of C and knew how to use it properly.

Complications termed *post-polio syndrome* occur in some individuals years after they've had polio. Whether extra C would ease the impact of the problem has not been determined. It would seem that those afflicted should consider trying it.

AIDS

Anecdotal evidence that 15 or more grams of C a day can suppress the signs and symptoms of AIDS prompted Pauling in the early 1980s to request funds for a clinical trial but he couldn't stir up any interest. Cathcart had tried also without success. In the fall of 1987 Pauling and Cameron presented evidence of the value of C to the President's Commission on AIDS but again were refused funds for a trial. The influential members of the commission preferred to leave the C stone unturned. Perhaps concern for the sick, if any, could not overcome the fear that C might be proven effective and result in a severe economic shock in certain circles. And no doubt the members had been influenced by the negative results of the cold trials that had used inadequate amounts of C.

Pauling's evidence, other than statements by physicians, consisted of the accounts of 6 men who had come to the Pauling Institute separately to tell how they controlled AIDS. Some had dropped out of experimental studies and some had decided to treat themselves from the start.

Common to all their self-treatments was the ingestion of 15 to 20 grams of C a day. Pauling told the Commission on AIDS that 4 of the 6 had had Kaposi's sarcoma. One still showed signs of it but he and the nurse who accompanied him stated that the sores were slowly disappearing. The man was strong enough to work as a carpenter, said not to be possible at that stage of the disease. Another man who'd had Kaposi's sarcoma was free of it but his T-cell count was still low. The count in the others was higher.

Cathcart wrote of his experience with AIDS patients plus that of about 90 others who had either self-treated or had been seen by other physicians who used C. Of the 12 Cathcart treated, only one died before the report was submitted for publication. He had been on chemotherapy and had had total body radiation. His veins were so frail that intravenous C could not be given [*Med Hypoth* 1984; 14:423-33].

Most AIDS patients can tolerate tremendous amounts of C by

mouth before diarrhea occurs, Cathcart noted. His doses, of ascorbic acid and its calcium, magnesium and potassium salts, were varied to suit the individual and taken in solution every hour or less. Starting doses ranged from 40 to 100 grams a day, as much as the bowel could tolerate. Persons having sickle-cell anemia, low G6PD or other rare conditions that react adversely to high doses of C should not be treated.

If oral doses were inadequate, intravenous C, 30 grams in a half liter of fluid, pH 7.4, were added. The amount of C could be doubled if patients had large veins. Those who were acutely ill were given 180 or more grams in vein over a 24-hour period, plus bowel-tolerance oral doses. Both he and Klenner mentioned that a gram of calcium gluconate daily should be given to prevent tetany during intravenous therapy with high-dose C.

Treatment also included elimination of intestinal parasites, yeast and other fungal infections that depress the immune system. Initially, the aggressive treatment may exacerbate symptoms due to a reaction to the load of inactivated viral and other organisms.

Cathcart gave a patient more than a half pound of C a day for 14 days. All symptoms were suppressed but no cure was achieved. In the early 1980s he felt that prolonged aggressive treatment begun at the start of HIV infection might clear the virus from the body. He advised that anyone exposed to it should take bowel-tolerance C indefinitely. Current knowledge suggests that it will be difficult to rid the body of the virus completely.

In *Vitamin C in Health and Disease* [Marcel Dekker, New York; 1997], Jariwalla and Harakeh state that C can "restore immune function in both viral and nonviral conditions linked to immunodeficiency." It protects cells targeted by viruses; stimulates the immune response; cuts viral DNA; inhibits viral enzyme activity; and may even prompt infected cells to die.

We wonder how those who hope the above information will never reach everyone infected with the virus can live with themselves.

8

How Much C Is Enough?

The statements in this chapter, or in any other, are not medical advice. They merely express opinions on how much C is advisable at different ages and under different conditions, assuming that an individual is well nourished, has normal iron status, no rare condition that is off-limits to high-dose C, and can take enough orally to counter a viral attack.

We have examined the trials that found C to be of little or no value in therapy---but found the trials themselves to be of little or no value. Seemingly proper but not really. In a word, deceptive. By those means, C has been unfairly discredited by the organizations we look to for guidance in matters of health. In general their guidance is good. But in regard to C as therapy for any condition other than scurvy they have been the ringmasters of a long-running fog-and-phony show.

Has the establishment failed us in the area of nutrition also? The adult nonsmoking RDA, now at 75 mg for women and 90 for men, had been kept at 60 mg or less for years, even as the results of studies suggested it should be raised. You'll recall the study of a group of dentists and spouses that found a *decline* in the average number of poor-health symptoms as the average intake of C *increased* toward 410 mg a day. And that worsening of arthritis in the knees can be retarded by taking 3 or more times the RDA. Also the report that optimum plasma C level requires 3 times the RDA. Aren't those findings reason enough to consider the RDA as far too low? We need more than just a borderline shield against scurvy. The C intake of our hunter-gatherer ancestors was nearly 400 mg a day. Why is it recommended that our current intake be so much less?

The standard argument against higher intake is that extra amounts are merely eliminated unchanged, doing nothing except creating expensive urine. This ignores the study that found extra C reduced the risk of urinary bladder cancer by inhibiting the formation of carcinogenic compounds there. And it may not have occurred to low-intake advocates that high urinary C may be Nature's way of preventing bladder infection. Or that C may have participated in chemical reactions in the body before being eliminated in its original state.

There's a double standard here. Large amounts of many other drugs are also found in the urine unchanged. Some are given with retardants to keep them in the body longer. According to the *Physicians Desk Reference,* more than half an oral dose of penicillin passes in the urine unchanged. [In the early days when it was scarce it was recovered and used again.] According to Canada's similar publication, 1988 edition, about 90% of the drug amantadine passes out unchanged. How's that for creating expensive urine! Would an advocate of low-C intake suggest that a dose of amantadine should be just as effective if it were reduced by 90%?

Critics have struggled mightily to convince the populace that taking extra C is folly. After a study on healthy persons found that little more than 2 grams of a dose can be absorbed, a group fed the data into a computer to show that a 20-gram dose is only marginally more available. Theoretical games of this sort are a hindrance to academic understanding of C. A healthy person would never take a 20-gram dose. A practicing physician, Cathcart, noticed that a sick body can absorb and utilize much more C than a well body, therefore we should consider practical experience as well as academic research when judging how much C is enough.

The question of how much an acutely ill person should take will be answered first because it probably interests the greatest number of readers. Suppose that a cold, flu, West Nile, or other viral disease attacks. Frankly, if you're young and healthy and colds don't bother much, skip the extra C---unless you want to experiment. But take bowel-tolerance doses as soon as possible to counter the more debilitating viruses. The amount to take, based on Cathcart's method, is 1 to 4 grams every 30 minutes ---enough to reach bowel-tolerance level quickly.

The key to successful use is to be aware of whether symptoms are easing off or coming on stronger. If they're stronger 20 minutes after dosing, one shouldn't wait another 10 minutes to take more C. If they're easing up after 30 minutes, dosing could be delayed 15 minutes or reduced a bit while close attention is paid to the direction symptoms are headed. For better judgment, avoid painkillers. And avoid laxative foods such as prunes so that the loose-stool signal comes from C alone. Taking C with orange juice and a fatty snack allows more absorption and utilization. The dose must be kept at bowel tolerance level as long as symptoms persist, then judiciously tapered down when the hint of diarrhea signals the body no longer needs as much C. If the thought of food brings on nausea, slowly sipping a C solution will do as well as long as the full dose gets down.

The above directions describe the ideal way of treating a viral illness. Unless a massive amount of beginner's luck prevails, the novice in C therapy will underdose and fail to benefit. Or will overdose and make frequent visits to the bathroom. Either way can cause a person to give up on C. Hang in there. Consider the search for dosing perfection a challenge---a sporting event in which the goal is to keep the sights on a moving target. In the beginning the target speeds away as symptoms worsen. Downing extra C slows it, stops it and reverses its direction so that less firepower is needed. Reduce the dose at that point but don't stop C completely, even if loose stools occur. Using less on the same schedule that eased the symptoms allows better control. If the choice is between bowel looseness and being sicker, most veteran dosers would choose the former.

If symptoms continue to worsen at bowel tolerance, either not enough C can be taken orally or the "bug" is bacterial, not viral. Intravenous C or antibiotics may be required. If antibiotics are used, some are more effective when extra C is taken also.

The ability to judge the intensity of an attacking disease comes with experience. Deciding on the dose and timing is also refined with practice. One might feel that taking more C only 20 minutes after the first dose is too soon. In some cases it is. The dose will not have peaked in the bloodstream for another hour or more. But the bloodstream is not the first performance arena for C---it just gets the most attention. As for what occurs in the gut, all we hear of is diarrhea. There may be benefits, more than we realize. The intestine is a convention site for bacterial toxins in illness and even in health. When they're absorbed we feel sick. Antitoxic C reduces them, allowing us to get through the day.

How much C is enough when we're cruising along in good health? There's no shortage of advice in this area. It ranges from the RDA of 75 mg to Pauling's 6,000 to 18,000 or more. A sampling: *Prevention* May 1996: 500 mg every 12 hours; Dec. 1996: 100 to 500 mg/day; Feb. 1997: 200 to 500 mg/day; *Wellness Letter* [Berkeley] May 1998: 250 to 500 mg/day; *American Health* Jan. 1999: 250 to 1,000 mg/day; *Healthy Living* Jan/Feb 1999: 500 to 5,000 mg/day; *Modern Maturity* May/June 1999: 500 mg/day. Klenner, you'll recall, favored a gram a day for each year a child is old up to age 10, when it is increased no more except during illness. The labels on some containers advise a gram a day for persons of age 12 or more.

It is difficult to justify giving healthy young teens a gram of C a day. Their tissues can remain saturated on a tenth of that amount. A decent diet will supply all the C required by that group. Age should be considered, then, when we advise on how much C is enough. The report mentioned on page 110 in which the C level of 20-year-old women averaged 1.1 mg/dl tells us they were doing very well without supplements. Men of that age were not, however. Their level of 0.8 is not enough to allow the formation of high quality collagen. Premium collagen requires a C level of at least 1 mg/dl, as the proteins used in its formation are in short supply when the level is at 0.9[1] At least 100 mg of C should be taken daily in order to maintain a higher level.

This is not to say we can't get along on substandard collagen. But if we demand high quality in our shoes and socks, our desire for the very best should at least extend to the glue that holds us together.   So many sprains and backaches may be due to substandard collagen.   You'll recall that the normal plasma C level listed in most books ranges from 0.4 to 1.5 mg/dl. If we're making poor collagen when the level is below 1, then *the lower half of the normal range is inadequate!*

Note this report: A man, 24, with a history of many infections developed an eye ulcer. His C level of 0.45 was in the normal range. His eye doctor put him on 3 grams of C a day while treating the ulcer. Afterward the man continued taking the dose and had no infections during a 2-year follow-up.[2] This report should send an important message to infection-prone individuals.

There's no reliable way to self-measure C level short of analyzing blood or plasma. Plasma C correlates with the number of seconds that pass before a drop of a particular dye on the tongue loses color but confounding variables make the test unreliable. Injecting dye just under the skin is also unreliable.

For practical purposes, simply taking extra C assures a high normal blood level.   How much extra? By now you probably suspect there are many answers. In general, healthy children and teen-agers whose diet includes potatoes [except French fries], fruit, vegetables and juices or drinks fortified with C are likely to have levels above 1 mg/dl. They have no need for supplements.

Nutritionists prefer to recommend fresh fruit and vegetables but canning or freezing doesn't remove all the C. In fact a half cup of boiled cabbage contains more C than a half cup of raw cabbage---not because boiling creates more C but because it reduces the bulk so that a half cup contains more cabbage. A red raw tomato contains 19 mg of C; stewed tomatoes of the same weight: 18 mg. Some less acid foods lose more C during processing. A raw peach contains 6 mg of C while one of the same weight canned has only 2 mg. Fresh is better. Potatoes, when baked or boiled retain a fair amount of C but have practically none when French fried or reconstituted from flakes. A fast-food baked potato supplies about 70 mg, a major portion of a teen's requirement. But they'd probably prefer a C-enriched drink.

Because our C level declines with age, increasing amounts must be taken to compensate. The great majority of individuals aged 30 to 55 probably would do better on a C intake that approaches the amount ingested by our ancient ancestors.

But if we feel well, isn't our C level adequate? Not always. A small amount of unhealthiness in some areas of the body can increase the need for C substantially. Consider periodontal disease. Many of us who appear to be in good health are afflicted. A recent study found that 2 grams of C a day along with a gram of calcium are required to improve this unhealthy condition around our teeth.[3]

If I were healthy and in the 30-to-55 age bracket, of average weight, I would aim for a C intake of 100 mg with each meal. I would not take more until sickness threatened, then I'd load in whatever it takes to overcome the problem---unless I'd decide to endure a bit of infection to stimulate antibody build-up.

The period between ages 55 and 60, or thereabouts, is a time of change. We're winding down. A good percentage of us may be able to continue taking 100 mg of C with each meal but others will need more. A decline in health can occur abruptly during the fifties. When the drop is evident it's time to consider raising the C intake---after making sure the iron status is normal.

Any increase should be substantial. Although one study found that *healthy women*, aged 60 to 80, need only about 2 mg of C per kilogram of body weight,[4] we shouldn't rely on studies of healthy individuals as a foundation for intake advice. The 2 milligrams per kilogram amount to a little less than a milligram per pound. A 140-pound woman, for example, would be advised to take 140 mg of C a day; a man the same weight: 210 mg.

My observations suggest that those intakes are not enough for the average senior citizen. The immune system is in decline, which will allow the flare-up of dormant viruses to cause all sorts of problems. The Epstein-Barr virus may potentiate the invasiveness of breast cancer.[5] Chickenpox virus causes shingles and can damage hearing. Hepatitis B and C viruses are linked to liver cancer [p63]. Hepatitis C virus is linked to an eye ulcer.[6]

A virus is associated with atherosclerosis[7] and the need for repeat angioplasty.[8] Rising viral antibodies during flare-ups of rheumatic disease suggest that high-dose C would be of value.[9] Measles virus has been linked to some cases of renal failure[10] and an outbreak of encephalitis.[11] Papilloma virus waits for low C and folic acid levels to weaken the barrier against uterine cervical cancer. Borna disease virus flares up to cause mental problems [p133]. The cold-sore virus causes Bell's palsy.[12] And if it is linked to Alzheimer's, then taking high-dose C would seem to be a logical attempt to prevent it, expecially for those who have close relatives with the disease.

We should never think that we don't harbor viruses. The carcinogenic Epstein-Barr virus, for example, persists in more than 90% of adults worldwide.[13]

A meager gram or two of C a day will not keep dormant viruses on hold for long. And they may not alert us to their activities with acute episodes. Their damage may be done so insidiously that we are not aware of the process until we notice a lower quality of life. My feeling is that the elderly who've had frequent viral attacks when young, or perhaps all oldsters, would fare better on a continuous high dose that approaches bowel tolerance. Not only to keep viruses in check; deaths were more numerous in the hospitalized elderly whose C level was low on entering.[14] A big problem with taking high-dose C, however, is in getting hospital personnel to maintain it, as we shall see.

154

Chapter 8 references

1   Buzina R, Aurer-Kozelj J, Srdak-Jorgic K, et al. Increase of gingival hydroxyproline by improvement of ascorbic acid status in man. *Int J Vit Nutr Res* 1986; 56:367-72

2   Foster C S, Goetzl E J. Ascorbate therapy in impaired neutrophil and monocyte chemotaxis. *Arch Ophthalmology* 1978; 96:2069-72

3   International Association for Dental Research 1998 annual meeting.

4   Itoh R, Yamada K, Oka J, et al. Sex as a factor in levels of serum ascorbic acid in a healthy elderly population. *Int J Vit Nutr Res* 1989; 59:365-72

5   Bonnet M, Guinebretiere J-M, Kremmer E, et al. Detection of Epstein-Barr virus in invasive breast cancers. *J Natl Cancer Inst* 1999; 91:1376

6   Wilson S E, Lee W M, Murakami C, et al. Mooren-type hepatitis C virus-associated corneal ulceration. *Ophthalmology* 1994; 101:736-45

7   Nieto F J, Adam E, Sorlie P, et al. Cohort study of cytomegalovirus infection as a risk factor for carotid intimal-medial thickening, a measure of subclinical atherosclerosis. *Circulation* 1996; 94:922-7

8   Epstein S E, Speir E, Zhou Y F, et al. The role of infection in restenosis and atherosclerosis: focus on cytomegalovirus. *Lancet* 1996; 348 (supp1):13s-17s

9   Salvarani C, Macchioni P, Boiardi L. Polymyalgia rheumatica. *Lancet* 1997; 350:43-7

10 Wairagkar N S, Gandhi B V, Katrak S M, et al. Acute renal failure with neurological involvement in adults associated with measles virus isolation. *Lancet* 1999; 354:992-5

11 Seppa N. Indian encephalitis traced to measles. *Sci News* 2000; 158:95

12 Murakami S, Mizobuchi M, Nakashiro Y, et al. Bell Palsy and herpes simplex virus: Identification of viral DNA in endoneurial fluid and muscle. *Ann Intern Med* 1996; 124:27-30

13 Young L S. Epstein-Barr-virus infection and persistence: a B-cell marriage in sickness and in health. *Lancet* 1999; 354:1141

14 Hunt C, Chakravorty N K, Annan G. The clinical and biochemical effects of vitamin C supplementation in short-stay hospital geriatric patients. *Int J Vit Nutr Res* 1984; 54:65-74

9

Odds & Ends

The "deadly" Ebola virus destroys so many blood vessel cells that most cases are fatal [*Science News* Aug. 5, 2000]. Vascular breakdown is also a first sign of scurvy. Cathcart noted that *acute induced scurvy* occurs when sickness quickly depletes the body's meager C reserve. Someday, someone treating Ebola disease will make the connection with scurvy and eliminate the word *deadly* by administering massive doses of C.

In southwestern U.S. a similar hemorrhagic fever is caused by Hantavirus. Doctors needn't go to Africa to become heroes. Nor should they suspect only exotic viruses when bleeding occurs. Several years ago a bright young adult in southeastern Michigan died of chickenpox. It was reported that transfused blood kept leaking from the veins. High-tech remedies could not help.

The thought of giving large doses of C doesn't arise in the minds of healthcare personnel. They've been brainwashed by the results of specious clinical trials that have blocked C from consideration as an antiviral, antitoxic substance. Marketing strategies are a boon in creating awareness of goods or services that raise the quality of life but a bane when used to mislead us.

The brains of oldsters with high C levels had healthier blood vessels, resulting in better mental function.[1] What about the ones who've reached 100 and are still dancing in the sunshine? Do they make their own C or just use it more efficiently than the rest of us? We'd think they've been running empty for years.

Scientists who've worked with guinea pigs note that they vary as much as 20-fold in the need for C. A very few, perhaps less than 1 in 1,000, can make their own C.[2,3,4] Do a few humans also have the ability? The question comes up occasionally, particularly with respect to infants.

Items in *Discover*, April 2000 and *Lancet* Aug.5, 2000 suggest that a virus may cause obesity in some persons. Certain viruses promote obesity in animals, leading to a look at humans. Sure enough, antibodies to a virus were found in 15% of 154 obese persons. The antibodies were not found in lean persons.

Cold sores and shingles have been triggered by vaccinations against other viruses.[5] The occurrence is rare but in the sick and old an attack by a dormant virus can be unpleasant. It has been reported that while 4% of persons under 20 have residual pain for more than a year after shingles, 70% of oldsters suffer pain.[6] Purpura, which may be due to low C, occurred in a man, 77, after he'd had a flu shot.[7] Taking more C might be protective.

The idea that Edgar Allen Poe died of rabies, not alcoholism, is supported by his lack of a boozy breath, difficulty in drinking water and alternating periods of delerium and lucidity, the last two being signs in rabid humans. C protects aginst rabies in guinea pigs. Of 50 animals not given C, 35 died. Of 48 injected with 100 mg of C per kilogram of body weight twice daily, 17 died,[8] about a 50% reduction achieved by a relatively low dose. The human equivalent, taken *orally*, is 14 grams twice a day for a person weighing 155 pounds. The time span is too long. Bowel-tolerance doses every 2 hours plus rabies shots as soon as possible after being bitten by a suspect animal would be better.

A question often asked is whether Ester-C, trademark for a patented calcium-ascorbate formula, is better than plain C. To those who believe brand names are better the answer is obvious. But to those who believe, for example, that the big name in aspirin is just another aspirin, brand names mean only higher price. A study at Arizona State University, on humans, published in the *Journal of the American Dietetic Association*, found that, despite all claims of superiority, Ester-C underperformed plain C a bit when C-equivalent doses were taken by 9 healthy persons.[9] Brand-name advertisers perform a valuable service, though, with their updated reports on the health advantages of a substance.

The study also found that the C with bioflavonoids commonly

found in vitamin stores, although slightly better absorbed than plain C, was not worth the extra cost. You'll recall reading in chapter 6 that 35% more C appeared in the bloodstream when in a citrus extract. Its concentration of flavonoids was much greater than the usual C complex found in stores, however.

Lupus erythematosus is an autoimmune disease---the type in which the immune system attacks body tissues. Victims have low C levels. Would extra C stimulate the immune system and lead to more tissue damage or would it stimulate repair of the damage and prevent further attacks? Extra C helps patients with multiple sclerosis, another autoimmune disease. A researcher in 1935 gave extra C to 2 lupus patients to increase its urinary excretion and reported no tissue damage. A patient with an acute episode was given 200 mg intravenously for 6 days, then a half liter of orange juice a day for a month with no report of tissue damage.[10] The kidneys may have been healthy. Sometimes they are not. Until more is known about the effect of C on this disease, patients should be wary.

Klenner, you'll recall, attributed his family's survival during the 1918 flu epidemic to tea brewed from the plant called *boneset*. At a later date he had the plant analyzed for C content and calculated that at one time the tea supplied 10 to 30 grams of the vitamin. The family must have consumed buckets of it.

Willow leaves, used by the Romans as well as by Native Americans, would have doubled the strength of the tea. Citing reliable sources, H.E. Sauberlich in *Vitamin C in Health and Disease* [Marcel Dekker, New York; 1997] listed the willow as having 465 mg of C per 100 grams of leaves. Boneset was not listed but a comparison made with an ascorbic acid dipstick shows willow leaves as having twice the concentration of C as boneset leaves. This is the wild willow that grows alongside streams. Weeping-willow leaves had about a third of the C contained in leaves of the wild willow.

I tested other plants and found red-pine needles equal to boneset leaves in C content. Dry brown needles, weighing less, had an even greater concentration. Dried flowers of boneset, also used in folk medicine, contained only a fourth of the C found in the leaves. The roots contained less. One wonders about the pioneers who sickened and died as the wagon trains rolled westward. They may have been on the brink of scurvy as they plodded on past the willows, unaware of the substance in the leaves that would have restored their health.

K.J. Carpenter in *The History of Scurvy and Vitamin C* [Cambridge University Press, Cambridge; 1986] wrote that scurvy hampered exploration of the far north. Seven volunteers were sent by Dutch merchants to spend the winter in Greenland in 1633. Relying on their best-laid plans and plenty of provisions, they felt they'd have no trouble waiting out the frigid winter. They made it through the worst of the cold but scurvy began to weaken them by March and progressed even though meat from the bears they shot would have supplied a small amount of C. The first man died in April. The rest died in early May.

Next september, 7 men arrived on the island of Spitzbergen to spend the winter. They were unable to find wild greens, nor were bears or small game available. Three died in January and all were dead by March. The accounts of other stranded groups in areas where game was available had happier endings, as most of the men, although quite ill, survived.

In 1743 four Russian sailors were stranded on the "remote eastern coast" of Spitzbergen with only an ax, knife, tinder, small kettle and a board with a nail and hook in it. They found an abandoned hut for shelter and managed to kill game with crude bows and arrows. They weren't able to make a fire but one of the men had wintered in frigid weather before. He told them to eat all the grass they could and had the fresh meat cut into bite-sized chunks so it would thaw in the mouth later. He also urged them to drink the blood of reindeer they killed. One man could not bring himself to do so. Scurvy progressively weakened him until he died. The other three managed to survive in the hostile climate for 6 years before they were rescued.

Rheumatoid arthritis "...has existed in North America for many thousands of years" but was unknown in Europe until after the return of Columbus and other explorers [*Lancet 9-18-99 p1026*].   This suggests that an infectious agent causes it. *Parvovirus B19* is suspected but it is also found in joints of well individuals. Either the finger is on the wrong "bug" or a susceptibility factor is involved. If a virus is the cause, then a long-term bowel-tolerance C regimen would be a logical treatment.

The regimen might also treat amyotrophic lateral sclerosis [Lou Gehrig disease]. According to the January, 2000 issue of *Neurology*, scientists have detected viral particles in the spinal cord of ALS patients. A 1982 paper had reported this but it was difficult to confirm at the time. *Good Housekeeping*, July 2001, notes that a patient in a cluster of cases in Texas took high doses of vitamin C, got better and returned to work for 10 years. The article also stated that doctors "don't advise anyone to try this unproven therapy." Since the therapy will never be proven [no money in it], patients who might be helped will continue to deteriorate. Every patient who can take high doses *should* try it. Not just a gram or two but 20 to 100 grams---bowel tolerance.

Tuberculosis and leprosy bacterial species are of the *Mycobacterium* genus. They do not produce toxin. A cousin in the genus, *Mycobacterium ulcerans*, does. Eventually it may be a greater healthcare burden than the other two.   This "flesh-devouring bacterium" of tropical regions around the world has attracted more attention lately. Its toxin spreads under the skin ahead of the bacterial advance, destroying deeper tissues, causing an ulcer [Buruli ulcer] that is difficult to treat. Pauling stated that C inhibits the growth of tuberculosis bacteria[11] and Cheraskin wrote that C destroys leprosy bacteria.[12] Perhaps C would be effective against their cousin *ulcerans* also, and against the toxin it produces. Healthcare personnel in countries that can't afford expensive remedies should look into the matter.

An ischemic stroke occurs when blood flow to part of the brain is stopped completely or reduced to a trickle by a clot in an artery that supplies the area. Brain cells die for lack of oxygen and glucose. The blood supply to the brain of a hibernating arctic ground squirrel is also reduced to a trickle, yet the brain cells survive. The animal's blood level of C is 4 times its level when not hibernating.

Researchers believe extra C is poised to reduce free-radical build-up that occurs during transition from deep sleep to an active life. In humans, some brain cells die when their blood supply is cut off---and some die as the flow resumes, presumably because of damage by free radicals. It has been suggested that this latter damage might be reduced by infusing C into a stroke patient during recovery.[13] [What are the odds on that ever becoming standard treatment?]

The article referenced above also reported that the brain of a sea turtle contains 5 times the amount of C found in human brains. The reason for so much is not known but guesses focus on free radicals again. A reduced oxygen supply to brains cells while turtles are submerged probably results in a surge of free radicals when turtles surface and oxygen is plentiful again.

It was mentioned in chapter 1 that extra C has been recommended for treating herpes since 1936. A man decided to try high doses after hearing of the old remedy from a relative who had attended one of my lectures. He wrote to confirm that C is as good as the expensive drug he had been using. A woman wrote that her mouth sores of 4 months duration cleared up when she took extra C on the advice of a physician. A man of 85 sent a color photo of himself that he'd had printed in quantity a few months before. The message under his smiling close-up stated that he was alive and well. He wrote that he'd taken 40 to 50 grams of C a day for several years.

Among the side effects of extra C explored in chapter 5 is its relationship with iron. The subject deserves frequent mention, as the rare harmful interaction between the two will become less rare as people raise their C intake beyond 500 mg a day. The *Wall Street Journal* alerted readers to age-related iron accumulation with two articles in 1992. In men, the body stores of iron begin to rise around age 20; in women around age 45. At 60, men have 6 times the iron stores they had at 20; women about 4 times, having dramaticaly increased storage after menopause. Also noted: about 1.4 million persons in the U.S. are genetically predisposed to hemochromatosis, an iron-overload condition. Most of them are not aware of it. A test of blood from more than 11,000 individuals indicated that about 1 in 200 Americans are prone to overload. Researchers have noticed a statistical correlation between excess iron and heart attack.

The body has no normal way to get rid of excess iron. Regular donation of blood helps. The thought has been expressed that one of the reasons a daily aspirin tablet helps prevent heart attacks is its tendency to cause minor gastrointestinal bleeding, thereby "donating" blood to the bowel for elimination.

As mentioned in chapter 5, the interaction between excess iron and high-dose C can damage organ tissue. Taking large amounts of the vitamin for a brief period of time to counter a viral attack should not be a hazard because the C is involved in zapping viruses, said to be a mutual-destruction event. But it should be emphasized that health-conscious individuals would do well to limit C intake to 500 mg a day until they know their iron status.

When we were in Oregon in August, 1990, my wife and I decided to drive south beyond San Francisco to visit the Pauling Institute, located in Palo Alto at the time. Dr. Pauling happened to be there. We sat and talked for a few minutes. When we rose to leave he rose also and walked us to the door. I had expected the 89-year-old man to struggle out of his chair and steady himself for a moment on a nearby desk before beginning a shaky step with an arthritic leg. None of that. He bounced up and strode with us like a 40-year-old. Perhaps he was anxious to get back to work. He was preparing for an upcoming symposium in Bethesda, sponsored by the National Institutes of Health.

162

The symposium was about biological functions of C and its relation to cancer. Several months after the event it was reported that, essentially, nobody showed up. Very few members of the sponsoring organization attended. Editors of all major medical journals were invited but only a representative from the AMA journal appeared. Ten years later we can detect a change for the better in attitudes about C. More reports of benefit are being printed in popular magazines. Extra C has been proved innocent in the kidney-stone area but it languished on death row for years before being exonerated. Better days are ahead.

References

1   Gale C R, Martyn C N, Cooper C. Cognitive impairment and mortality in a cohort of elderly people. *Br Med J* 1996; 312:608-11
2   Odumosu A, Wilson C W M. Metabolic availability of vitamin C in the guinea pig. *Nature* 1973; 242:519-21
3   Ginter E. Ascorbic acid synthesis in certain guinea pigs. *Int J Vit Nutr Res* 1976; 46:173-9
4   Williams R J, Deason G. Individuality in vitamin C needs. *Proc Natl Acad Sci USA* 1967; 57:1638-41
5   Walter R, Hartmann K, Fleisch F, et al. Reactivation of herpesvirus infections after vaccinations? *Lancet* 1999; 353:810
6   Kost R G, Straus S E. Postherpetic neuralgia --- pathogenesis, treatment and prevention. *N Engl J Med* 1996; 335:32-42
7   Patel U, Bradley J R, Hamilton D V. Henoch-Schonlein purpura after influenza vaccination. *Br Med J* 1988; 296:1800
8   Banic S. Prevention of rabies by vitamin C. *Nature* 1975; 258:153-4
9   Johnston C S. Luo B. Comparison of the absorption and excretion of three commercially available sources of vitamin C. *J Am Diet Assoc* 1994; 94:779-81
10 Finkle P. Observations on excretion of vitamin C in some vascular diseases. *Proc Experi Biol Med* 1935; 32:1163-4
11 Pauling L. *How to Live Longer and Feel Better*, P 167 [Avon, New York; 1986]
12 Cheraskin E, Ringsdorf W M Jr., Sisley E L. *The Vitamin C Connection* p 47 [Bantam Books, NewYork; 1983]
13 Travis T. Chilled brains. *Science News* 1997; 152:364-5

10

Personal C
Experience

Only a few individuals have written of their own benefit from taking large amounts of C for years. Klenner wrote that on 10 to 20 grams a day the brain was clearer, the mind more active, the body less weary and the memory more retentive. Sherry Lewin, author of the 1976 book *Vitamin C: Its Molecular Biology and Medical Potential*, normally took 2 grams a day. Earlier, he had been skeptical of the idea that extra C is beneficial but began to take 50 mg a day because his wife thought the pill might relieve symptoms of his frequent colds. Later, she substituted 1,000-mg pills, saying she couldn't get the smaller ones. Not wanting to throw them away, he used them---and had less misery from colds, moreso when he took a gram an hour. He also noticed fewer of the symptoms that had preceded a heart attack in 1967.

Albert Szent-Gyorgyi, who first isolated C, didn't write of his dose but a magazine article stated that a gram a day was his usual dose except during a bout with pneumonia at age 84, when he took 8 grams daily. He died at 92 in 1986, having lived a very interesting life. He did write of that [ref 8, chapter 6].

Biochemist Irwin Stone wrote that his daily dose was 3 to 5 grams. Another authority takes 5 grams a day. When we talked via phone he seemed reluctant to reveal the amount. There's a feeling that high-dosers are shelved alongside those sincere folks who tell of having been beamed aboard a spaceship. But a scientist I talked with did not hesitate to mention his daily dose of 36 grams. When asked why so much he replied that he'd been subject to infections all his life until he tried C in various amounts. He found the most effective amount to be his bowel-tolerance limit---36 grams.

Linus Pauling, who took other vitamins and minerals also, began taking 3 grams of C daily at about age 70. He raised the intake periodically until reaching his tolerance limit of 18 grams. More was taken when ill or if his schedule required an increase. He died at 93 in 1994. Cathcart wrote in 1992 that in 22 years he had taken about 361 kilograms of C. It averages out at about 45 grams a day but, like Pauling, he started with lower doses and as tolerance developed increased the intake to maintain benefits.

Cathcart and Pauling can be considered true experts on C because they have taken high doses for years, raising the amount whenever necessary. Those who have not had this personal experience cannot know all about C. They're like the early mapmaker who could only print HERE BE DRAGONS in the blank areas where he'd never been.

High-dose C is indeed a blank area in the medical literature. No academic effort has been made to explore it---DRAGONS!!! No doubt this is due to lack of funding. It is unfortunate because some of the major benefits of extra C occur only at the high doses that healthcare personnel ignore. Information about those "astronomical amounts" is available to the public only by hearsay and the few writings of high-dosers.

Perhaps you'll develop a better understanding of the nature of C if I relate my own experience far beyond the RDA horizon. In early 1986, at age 69, while browsing in a bookstore I happened to come across Pauling's new book, *How to Live Longer and Feel Better*, mentioned earlier. I was aware that he had written books on the common cold and flu but hadn't read them. Like most people, I felt that if vitamin C was so effective it would be used regularly by the medical community. Dentists, like physicians, believe the wellspring of all reliable health information is located in the university nesting areas where they fledged.

The book's title was appealing, however, because during the previous summer I had begun to feel my age. A neck muscle developed a soreness after I'd hoed the garden. It persisted all summer, demanding a wince every time I turned my head. Hauling a few loads of dirt in the wheelbarrow would bother my back for a week. Sometime earlier a slow fungus had invaded my toenails, thickening them. Then the same species, or a relative, began to spread a dry non-itching ruddy sheet slowly across the top of my left foot, just behind the toes. Another relative of the clan found a home in my left ear, requiring a bit of medication about every 4 or 5 days to control the itching. A black slash, about the size of a grain of rice, appeared in the visual field of my right eye. And weariness came on sooner than usual, a most disappointing curse to one who revels in slowly changing the landscape by the regular application of physical labor.

All that, yet I had been taking 500 mg of C a day plus extra vitamins and minerals for several years.

In his book, Pauling advised taking from 6 to 18 grams of C a day. *Spoonfuls!* Like nearly everyone else at the time, I thought such doses were toxic! To make sure the amount was not a misprint I visited the medical library nearby to read a few of the papers referenced in the book.

Assured that a 6-gram dose wouldn't be fatal, but still somewhat apprehensive, I took 4 half-gram tablets after breakfast one day, was still breathing at noon so took another 4 after lunch and a third such dose after the evening meal. No diarrhea or other reactions occurred. At the time I wasn't aware that about 20% of those who take more than a gram or two would develop intestinal gas or cramps or some other nuisance reaction.

The first benefits were noticeable within a week: the ear stopped itching. Apparently the larger dose had sounded reveille to the immune system. And I felt stronger, as if I could tool around with the wheelbarrow all day as soon as the ground was free of frost. Other benefits followed. The fungus on my foot that had been advancing like a giant ameba began to retreat. In 4 weeks there was on sign of it. The thickened toenails responded slower but eventually slimmed down to almost normal. And in a few months I could no longer detect the black slash in my right visual field.

Best of all, a "spastic gut" condition, a bothersome thing for years, vanished. Now why would extra C, which causes cramps in some individuals, rectify a condition in my innards that was itself a cause of cramps? Is C neutralizing a continuous flow of toxins generated by bacteria? Or is it controlling a remnant viral population, the measles virus, for example? According to some reports, measles virus can persist in the gut for years. Whatever, being rid of the nuisance meant that I could eat beans and salads without experiencing discomfort that once had caused me to feel that such food was fit only for rabbits. I felt better than I had in years, assured that the fountain of youth bubbled up from an aquifer of vitamin C solution.

If this narrative were set to music the sound would be light and bouncy, the kind that would prompt a party of oldsters to dance around a picnic table loaded with goodies and C pills while radiating all the frenetic joy captured in beer commercials. ...Up to this point. Then the music would turn ominous, as when the wolf comes to blow the piggie's house down.

Ten weeks after the start of the regimen the ear began to itch again. Doubts about the permanence of benefits began to brew. Those ongoing horror stories about kidney stones and dire toxicities alleged by the anti-C mafia added to the concern. From the beginning they hadn't completely vanished from my thoughts. I considered abandoning the regimen. Meanwhile, I had been visiting the medical library regularly to learn more about the vitamin and why it generated so much controversy.

The more I read, the more I came to realize that C was being treated unfairly by the system. Although there were legitimate concerns, bias was evident and the footprints of a marketing strategy could be detected in the literature. A veteran cynic might suspect that certain bad guys in black didn't care to have people feeling so well that markets for expensive drugs would shrink. But I was no veteran. I had only begun to read.

My decision to continue the 6-gram regimen was influenced

by two factors: First, I didn't care to rekindle my feeling of the the previous summer that infirmity was fast approaching; second, if Pauling could take 18 grams a day I should be able to take 8. I raised to that amount. The ear itch vanished. It returned again about 10 weeks later. I raised my intake to 10 grams a day. By then I had adopted an attitude that if being a victim of toxicity was to be my lot it would warn others and provide critics with the pleasure of reporting a casualty of the "fad" of high-dosing on vitamin C.

Fortunately, I had no reactions at any time. If I had known at the start that extra C is a hazard in iron overload, however, I would not have begun the regimen without first having my iron status determined. Even though the hazards of extra C are quite rare, advocates of high intakes should be sure to mention them. Many individuals who take warfarin, for example, are probably not aware that more than a gram of C per day might reduce the effectiveness of their dose.

The ear itch kept returning about every 10 weeks and I kept increasing my daily intake by 2 grams, wondering if the upward ratcheting would ever end. Finally, at 16 grams a day, the itch failed to return on schedule. This is a good demonstration of the tolerance effect---the build-up of enzymes by the body to handle the large amount and a probable change in gut bacteria to species that relish the vitamin.   In my case, the effects of both were overwhelmed each time I raised the dose, allowing a little more C, probably not more than a few milligrams, to reach areas where it bestowed a benefit.

A person who lacks the convenience of an itch as a guide to adequate dosing must look for other symptoms that announce the need to increase intake. It could be a difficult call. Some benefits appear so slowly, and might fade as slowly, that attributing them to C would be guesswork. Before I began the high-dose regimen my shoulder, left knee and right hip joints twinged a bit from arthritis. They don't now, 16 years later, but the condition resolved so slowly that I can't remember when the improvement was first noticed. And my neck vertebrae grated as if in gravel whenever I turned my head but at some undetermined time the "gravel" converted to fine sand.

Before I ever thought of taking extra C I had noticed recurring discomfort in the right abdomen that suggested a gas pocket in the gut. It turned out to be a stone in the ureter, the tube that drains a kidney into the bladder. I had been on the C regimen for several months before learning of it. If the condition hadn't bothered before high dosing I would have blamed C. Six years later a stone in the same spot bothered again. It was not caused by C either. In both cases my poor sense of thirst was at fault. I hadn't been drinking coffee, tea, soft drinks, beer or even much water. The first stone should have been fair warning but a second was needed to make me change my ways.

Now I take more fluids plus a 100-mg tablet of magnesium citrate-B6 3 times a day. A study reported in 1974 found that magnesium and a small amount of vitamin B6 reduced stone recurrence dramatically [*J Urol* 1974; 112:509]. No third stone has shown up in the 10 years since the second stone occurred. When checked recently, my blood oxalate level was in the normal range, slightly above the midpoint. My uric acid level was slightly below the middle of the normal range.

While I was building up to the 16-gram regimen I had no colds, just some sniffles about every third or fourth year, presumably when diminishing antibodies to the viruses needed boosting. I had a history of enduring 6 to 8 cold sores every winter. Since taking high-dose C I've had a total of only 2. One occurred after hard work exhausted me. The second followed a bout with the 1994 flu. I had failed to raise my dose at the first hint of attack, thinking the vague symptoms were due to a stray cold virus and would soon go away.

To experiment, I'd had no flu shots between 1988 and 1997, hoping to lure a virus into combat. One took the bait in 1990 and was quickly vanquished with 4 grams of C an hour. By hour 20 all flu symptoms were gone. An experienced doser would have reduced C intake at hour 21 but I didn't. Only then did diarrhea occur. The experience---the realization that 80 grams of C could be swallowed in less than a day during an illness without a change in bowel habits---is an epiphany that would convert even a hard-core doubter into an advocate of vitamin C.

The foregoing was my experience with the 1990 flu. The 1994 bug that ambushed me had advanced too far to be aborted. When I realized my mistake, the mean reputation that preceded that year's flu suggested the ordeal would be long and debilitating. I couldn't block it. I could only minimize the symptoms with frequent dosing after first downing fatty food, usually canned salmon, ice cream, or peanut butter on bread, sometimes as often as every 20 minutes. The disease ran a benign course. No misery; just a lazy feeling for two days and a bit of diarrhea from overdosing. Compared to previous bouts with flu in past years, this was cake.

My father had a growth in the crease alongside his nose that had reached the size of a blueberry. It was a basal-cell carcinoma. He had been painting the cracked-open surface with iodine. When he came to visit he resisted making an appointment to have it removed until I showed him a picture of a man who had lost a quarter of his face to the scalpel before every last cell of the cancerous "rodent ulcer" had been eliminated.

The same type of growth had started in the same location on my face. Not long before I began high-dosing with C a little red dot appeared in the center of the dark growth. I had been watching for signs of breakdown and scabbing that would suggest it was the same growth my father had. Still I didn't think of removing it. When I was taking 8 or 10 grams of C a day the growth began to recede. A year later only a raised freckle marked the spot. Klenner wrote that he had eliminated several basal-cell growths by applying a paste of C. I tried his method on the freckle for a week, until the area was quite inflamed from the acidic nature of the paste. After the redness subsided the freckle remained.

Next, a similar growth appeared on the other side of my face in the typical location, this one after I'd taken high-dose C for 10 years. It too followed the same pattern of steady expansion, then fading. At present, not even a freckle remains of either. I think they both would have continued as basal-cell carcinomas but can't be sure as no biopsy was done. They were not warts. Some warts can be removed quickly by applying a C paste twice a day. Others are more resistant but eventually succumb also.

Each of my closest relatives---mother, father and brother--- suffered from shingles when in their 70s. To date, thanks to C, I'm sure, I've not had the disease. Prior to 1986 when a physician friend was afflicted with shingles as mentioned on page 1 [case WC], I hadn't known that C could treat it. Since then my knowledge of the vitamin's antiviral nature has expanded somewhat. A few years later he phoned about a bridge partner who had just developed the typical blisters on his abdomen. I suggested the man take 3 or 4 grams of C after each meal. My physician friend, wary of such a massive amount, advised his bridge partner to take only 5 grams a day. It helped for a time but the inadequate dose provided no sustained relief.

Specious clinical trials plus constant mention of toxicity lock most physicians into the belief that C has little therapeutic value and is dangerous in high doses. Any treatment not "evidence based" is looked upon as questionable. Deceptive trials have denied C the benefit of good evidence, therefore it is classed as alternative therapy, interpreted by many to mean quackery.

This pervasive bias against alternative therapy has elicited some interesting comments on the subject from establishment members. *The Lancet* prints a column in which questions are asked of prominent physicians and educators. Questions such as who was your most influential teacher; what is your greatest love [or pleasure, fear, regret, etc]; how do you relax; how do you want to die and other probes intended to bring out the essence of

the individual. A pair of questions often answered: What alternative therapies have you tried? Did they work?

Some answers: "Absolutely not!" [7-1-98].   "Alcohol."
[7-25-98].   "You must be joking!" [10-3-98].   "None. But I
have spent...time defending the right of...zanies, oddballs and
fanatics to pursue their dubious visions of healing." [10-17-98].
"I haven't tried any alternative therapy and it has worked so far."
[10-31-98].   "I'm saving alternative therapies until I succumb to
an alternative disease." [11-14-98].   "None. If they worked
they'd no longer be alternative." [12-19/26-98].

Ponder whether the editor would have printed this answer: "If
certain alternative therapies had been evaluated in fair trials they
would no longer be alternative."

We shouldn't omit comments by those who were not so
biased that curiosity was stifled. Examples: "About a million.
Currently flaxseed oil---and who knows, maybe this one will
work!" [2-6-97].   "Broccoli, soy milk, green tea. I'll find out in
50 years." [5-1-99].   One felt echinacea worked [5-23-98].
Another favored vitamins and minerals [1-2-99].   And one was
so bold as to admit that he'd tried C for a cold but wasn't sure it
worked [8-1-98].

A gentleman began his reply with: "A certain disregard, or
even contempt, for our minor ailments is a therapy that is not
used often enough" [1-9-99].

Be aware, however, that pinpointing the fine line between a
minor and a major ailment is not always easy. To guess wrong
could be disastrous.

A problem I encountered arose because of contempt for a
minor ailment along with an inability to locate the line between
it and a major illness. I felt so well armored with high-dose C
that no disease could reach me. I'd had no pain at all from a
prostate "reaming" at age 70 while the groans of others in
adjoining rooms were somewhat unsettling. Whoever said C is
absolutely super as a painkiller was correct [at least for that
condition but a stone in the ureter is another matter].   Ten years

later, still taking 16 grams a day, I continued to feel great. Sure, the aging hulk was lower in the water but had no list to port or starboard.

The ear had begun to itch occasionally, however. I increased the daily dose to 18 grams, then to 20 soon afterward. The need for so much so soon should have alerted me, I suppose, that something more than normal aging was increasing the demand.

The spring of 1997 marked the beginning of this increased requirement, when, after I'd turned 80, thinking I was 40, I decided to extend a concrete driveway alongside the garage. I used a mixer because the job was too small and access too limited for delivery by truck. After starting, one must continue working at a concrete job until it's finished, come hell or Murphy's law, the equivalent, which is sure to kick in. Inhaling cement dust that hung in the air like fog during the windless day while I pitched shovelful after shovelful of ingredients into the hungry mixer was no great comfort either. But I was only working beyond the point of exhaustion, as was my custom, confident that high-dose C would bounce the body back to normal in a day or two.

The bounce-back was not 100%. Inhaled cement dust may have limited it. Alkaline particles could have weakened lung tissue and invited infection. In midsummer, after a few more hard-work periods to show contempt for the minor ailment, pneumonia became a threat. Six different antibiotics in succession failed to banish the feeling that the lungs were not up to par.

I visited a pulmonary specialist. While pondering the results of a standard checkup plus my answers to questions, he wondered whether I could tell the difference between bronchitis, heartburn, hunger and a gas pocket. His diagnosis: gastroesopha-geal reflux---heartburn. On thinking about it, heartburn could be expected because of my routine: a snack plus 4 grams of ascorbic acid just before bedtime. Topping off a little food with an acid drink is not a good idea. Along with the usual advice for handling heartburn, the doctor prescribed cisapride, trade name Propulsid, to promote movement of food out of the stomach.

Thirty days later, on the morning before a scheduled return visit, I wakened with a swollen left ankle. The sign always appears in the left ankle first, it is said---the sign of heart failure. The combination of continual overexertion, infection and heart-burn had resulted in a serious problem. Antibiotics and cisapride may have been factors also The drug book *PDR* begins its information about cisapride with a warning that heart damage might occur. Due to a lapse in alertness I had not read the warning before taking the drug. Later the *Wall Street Journal* [6-30-98] announced that the FDA had issued a strong warning against routine use of it. Finally, in March 2000, the drug was removed from the market because of a number of reported deaths.

The pulmonary specialist had me wheeled to the nearby hospital. Now here is why I'm relating this experience: nearly everyone will be hospitalized sooner or later, including those who take extra C, so be aware of this hazard: *The hospital staff may not give you the amount of C you have been accustomed to taking!* When the nurse, a man, checked me over I told of my high dose and the rebound effect if it is discontinued. It went over like small talk. Later a resident physician examined me. I spoke of the need for at least 4 grams of C after each meal. He smiled, the patronizing kind a mother would use when a kiddie tells of a bunny that goes lippity-lippity down a garden path.

The evening medication included two little pills, probably 100 mg each. The nurse wouldn't say. I complained. He said we could talk about in the morning. When he came in at six in the morning I was putting on my clothes.

"I'm getting out of here," I said.

"No you're not."

"The hell I'm not! You can't keep me here!"

He left. The day-shift resident physician entered, a bright young lady I'd met before in the specialist's office. I thought she would understand the problem but the standard bias against C governed her approach.   Although many medications are not reduced abruptly, she didn't feel that C is in that class. Nothing I could say would change her mind and she said I might die if I left the hospital.

I might die if I stayed there! I thought. I left.

The lesson here is that a high-doser who is hospitalized risks a compounding of the illness due to the rebound effect. Abrupt stoppage of even a gram of C can damage tissue in some persons. Note the retinal hemorrhages a diabetic developed [p 122]. Note that disease afflicted millions when the potato shortage deprived the people of Ireland of their daily gram [p 90].

I mourn the loss of a friend whose gram of C a day was stopped abruptly when pneumonia put him in hospital at 70. Perhaps he wouldn't have survived anyway but lack of his usual dose further reduced his chances, which, in my opinion, would have increased substantially by intravenous infusion of 100 grams a day. Although some hospitals recognize a patient's need for maintaining an adequate C level, others regard the taking of supplements as interfering with their own therapy. It's been said that a collection of ideas about C from the latter institutions would constitute a major exhibit on *The Antiques Roadshow.*

Cathcart advised high dosers to carry a wallet card to alert hospital personnel of the need for continuing the dose. In my case a card would have been useless. Better to have a friend who can make sure the directions on the card are followed. If the usual daily dose continues to be disregarded.......there's enough evidence in the medical literature to support a conclusion that the patient is not receiving proper care.

I checked into another hospital a week later. This time I brought along a week's supply of C in my shaving kit. Taking it without being observed was no problem. How sad that one must resort to stealth in order to avoid the risk of a prolonged hospital stay. Instead of rejecting C it should be infused routinely, as hospital patients are known to have low C levels.

The supply of C to primates in zoos receives better attention.

Because the ACE inhibitor I was given tends to make one cough, my frequent whoops were attributed to the drug until my temperature began to rise. The pneumonia, now definite, was cleared up by azithromycin, a drug I hadn't used. I was discharged feeling much better. The heart ejection fraction which was at 20% is much higher now, more than 4 years later.   I have added acetyl-L-carnitine, alpha lipoic acid, Co-Q 10, flax oil, and more vitamin E and folic acid to my regimen. Although I don't make unreasonable demands on the heart anymore, I can push the mower around for an hour without becoming winded.

The bronchial infection which appeared to trigger all the later events has returned 3 times. Extra C can be of great benefit in many situations but obviously not for this condition. A 5-day course of azithromycin cleared the infection the first time. Several months later when it returned it was routed with only 4 capsules of echinacea, one after each meal.   Only 3 capsules were needed when the infection threatened a third time.

Tha above paragraph was written as a lead-in to another warning: You'll recall from chapter 3 that echinacea prompts certain white cells to release tumor necrosis factor and that this may do more harm than good in patients with certain diseases. I've read that heart failure is one of them. Echinacea should be used as little as possible by those of us with that condition.

A hard-core critic of extra C might say, "Aha! You took too much and it damaged your heart!"

Not so. During recovery I raised my intake to 36 grams a day and afterward reduced it to 28 grams, not the 20 I had been taking at the beginning of the problem. I have raised it since to about 32 grams.

I don't measure doses precisely; just take a high-rounded teaspoon of ascorbic acid powder in about a quarter cup of tomato-vegetable juice after breakfast; the same amount in a half cup of orange juice at noon; and again that much in a half cup of cranberry cocktail-grape juice after the evening meal.   About an hour before bedtime, after a snack I take 2 rounded teaspoons of the bitter C---calcium ascorbate powder---in a half cup of water. When weighed recently, a day's dose amounted to a little over 32 grams.

C is not a cure-all. It hasn't quieted the mild ringing in my ears that began in the 1960s. I didn't expect it to. But I did hope it would prevent the leg cramps that occasionally disturb my sleep. It didn't. My current strategy is to stretch the calf muscles for a few minutes before bedtime. Nor does C prevent the "winter itch" we oldsters complain about. And it was of no value in preventing the annoying cracks in my finger tips that occurred every winter---but vitamin E is preventive. Not at the usual 400 units a day, however. In my case no cracks have appeared during the last 3 winters while taking at least 2,400 units a day. C regenerates E. They work well together.

There is good reason to believe that C plus a healthy lifestyle can prolong life. In addition to the findings noted on page 140, a report in *The Lancet*, August 11, 2001, p472-3, states that white-cell telomeres are shorter in patients with atherosclerosis, comparing with controls 8.6 years older, on average. Telomere "caps" on the ends of chromosomes are said to determine life span. They shorten over the years as new cells are produced.

If extra C, proper diet and exercise can prevent the diseased condition it seems that we wouldn't lose those years. Hypothetically, any other chronic infection will shorten life in the same manner, as accelerated production of white cells during infection causes them to use up their quota of telomeres sooner than normal. Then we run out of infection-fighting white cells.

The late William Saroyan wrote that he knew people must die but hoped God would make an exception in his case. God didn't. Nor can we expect C to change the rules. But we *can* expect C to help prolong life up to the point allowed by our genetic program. And when someone finds a way to lengthen telomeres so that it leads to standing-room only on the planet, extra C should also make a long life more bearable.

Some readers may decide to start high-dosing on C after reading of its many benefits. Good---but remember the conditions in which rare side effects are more than just a nuisance. People with poor kidney function or who've had part of the upper intestine removed may have a problem with oxalate. Those on anticoagulants should have the clotting picture monitored if taking more than a gram of C a day. Anyone with paroxysmal nocturnal hemoglobinuria, G6PD deficiency or iron overload should read chapter 5 again. Do not begin a long-term program of high-dose C without first determining the body's iron status. If low G6PD is suspected, it is better to start by increasing C intake by a gram a day while watching for brown urine that signals destruction of red cells. Couples with the trait should beware of gene roulette at conception that can design a baby with much lower G6PD.

Unless one is committed to becoming a slave to a dosing schedule it makes no sense to begin a high-dose regimen. It is said that about half of those who take prescription drugs do not take them as directed. They might fail to take C properly also. Haphazard dosing is worse than no dosing. Doses should be taken regularly, with no habitual skipping. And remember the hazard of a hospital stay, where there's danger of being deprived of the high dose by uninformed or biased hospital staff.

During her preparation for surgery, friend Alice mentioned that she takes 15 grams of C a day. She was asked why and who advised such a massive dose.

"Started it myself. It keeps my lungs clear," she replied.

"Prescribed by doctor Alice!" sniffed a physician who overheard the conversation.

An attitude of that sort is hazardous to high-dosers' health. Illegal drug users get more respect.

Currently there's not much encouragement to use extra C by most members of the healthcare professions. For too long they've been misled by deceptive clinical trials. The mindset can't be changed overnight. Members of the professions should look to the source of the problem: journal editors. Their refusal to publish the results of deceptive studies would go a long way toward allowing C a fair appraisal as a therapeutic substance. Editors as a group should have the courage to tell advertisers to take their business elsewhere if the content of the journals doesn't please them. What could advertisers do? Just what they do now---continue to advertise even as journals publish papers that demonstrate the superiority of a competing prescription product.

Journal editors do appear to be interested in dispensing information that would further the wellbeing of people everywhere---but only if the information doesn't compete with a drug company's product. I've written more than a dozen letters to various editors, pointing to evidence that C is of value in treating certain conditions. All that comes of the effort is a form-letter reply to the effect that there's no room to include the information in the journal. The following is an example:

June 2, 2001

Editor, *Lancet*:

Sir---In the May 26 issue David McNamee wrote of a new antivenom.[1] The use of 6 to 12 vials at U.S. $775 per vial puts it out of reach of victims in countries that need it most. Papers in the medical literature point to ascorbic acid (or ascorbate) as a less expensive way to detoxify venoms. In 1937 Jungeblut, citing 18 references, wrote that ascorbic acid inactivated every toxin it had been tested against.[2] In 1952 W. J. McCormick stated that he had "obtained rapid recovery in a case of scorpion sting by a single intravenous injection of 1,000 mg."[3] In 1971 F.R.Klenner wrote of countering highland mocassin venom with intravenous doses of the substance. He preferred it to antivenom.[4] Black-widow spider bites were treated effectively also.[5] In 1993 Dettman, Kalokerinos and Dettman[6] referred to a 1947 paper in a Colombian journal[7] (unavailable here) which detailed emergency treatment of 3 snakebite cases with 2 grams of ascorbic acid in vein. A "very favorable response" was seen immediately after the first injection. Follow-up injections, if necessary, were given every 3 hours.

New drugs are a boon where there's a need but replacing an excellent inexpensive substance with an exotic, toxic and expensive substitute is greedy, callous and ridiculous.

1   McNamee D. Tackling venomous snakebites worldwide. *Lancet* 2001;357:1680.
2   Jungeblut C W. Further observations on vitamin C therapy in experimental poliomyelitis. *J Experi Med* 1937;66:459-77.
3   McCormick W J. Ascorbic acid as a chemotherapeutic agent. *Arch Pediat* 1952;69:151-55.
4   Klenner F R. Observations on the dose and administration of ascorbic acid when employed beyond the range of a vitamin in human pathology. *J Appl Nutr* 1971;23:61-88.
5   Klenner F R. The black widow spider. *Tristate Med J* 1957;Dec:15-18
6   Vitamin C, p 422. *Dettman G C, Kalokerinos A, Dettman I.* (Frederick Todd, Melbourne; 1993.)
7   Perdoma H. Snake venom and vitamin C. *Revista de la faculatad de Medicina (Bogota).* 1947;15:769-72.

Sincerely, etc.

Although the new substance counters only bites from rattlers and related snakes, I hoped to get in a word about C. In reply, a letter stated that the journal had no room for the information.

It's understandable; snakebite victims who need 6 to 12 vials of the antivenom at $775 per vial would pour from $4650 to $9,300 into the pharmaceutical revenue pipeline. Vitamin C would provide relief for from $5 to $20. As long as information about the cheaper method does not circulate a tremendous cash flow *does* circulate---from the manufacturer to the journal in ads, generous salaries to editors and substantial income to journal owners. No one should object to financial incentives when a needed service is provided. But to milk the sick by promoting expensive treatments while suppressing information about cheaper alternatives is akin to robbery.

C has few defenders against the disreputable acts of those who gain from hammering on it. Even the editors of health magazines for the general public take care not to praise the versatility of C too much. They too have their eyes on ad revenue as well as access to research nuggets, those cutting-edge treatments that are regular items in news reports these days.

I checked for a listing of vitamin C, ascorbic acid or ascorbate in the indexes of more than a dozen virology textbooks shelved in a nearby medical library. Only one referred to the vitamin, with the comment that mention was made only because of public awareness of its promotion for treatment of the common cold, for which it was not shown to be beneficial. In the eyes of the authors of those books, the supreme oracles of all things viral, vitamin C as an antiviral substance does not exist. One would think they had no knowledge at all of the studies done at universities in Switzerland or the reports of Klenner, Cathcart, Stone, Murata and many others. No wonder the healthcare community is unaware of its value.

Readers should question every negative statement about vitamin C because most members of the pharmaceutical-medical complex have a financial stake in discrediting it. They would have us believe that our welfare is their first concern but we have seen otherwise. They cannot be trusted. We are left with the impression that the C genie must be kept in the bottle at all costs---to those who are ill.

If not in stores, this book can be ordered at $4.95 postpaid from Service Press, Box 130104, Ann Arbor, MI 48113. Allow 2 weeks, more or less, for delivery. Add $2.50 if faster Priority Mail shipping is desired. No shipping in November & December. No shipping after October 2005.